WHAT PEOPLE ARE SAYING ABOUT

MIDDLE AGE BEAUTY

Middle Age Beauty is wise and ... es the
reader to see herself in t ... ways.
Machel Shull writes from ... rney
with great generosity. Any ... inner peace
will love this book.
Luanne Rice, #1 *New York Times* Bestselling Author of *Little Night*
and Author of 31 novels

I am adding *Middle Age Beauty* to my selected few bedside
books. With Machel's light to guide us home to our true beautiful
selves, we can celebrate being the hero of our own story.
MJ Rolek, Zen Life Coach and Author of *Mental Fitness, Complete
Workouts for Body, Mind, and Soul*

Machel Shull has compiled a treasure of secrets, insights and
practical tips that are both inspiring and instructional. She has
artfully drawn from her experience, wisdom, gift of writing, and
most of all courage, to create the valuable gift that is a must-read
for middle aged women who have ever questioned their true
beauty.
Dr. Anthony F. Smith, Co-founder and Managing Director of
Leadership Research Institute, Bestselling Author and Professor
of Leadership

Ms. Shull shares a wonderful personal account of maintaining a
'natural' position of beauty. In an age of new treatments,

methods and synthetics, she sticks to the basics of how using nature is perhaps the best way to preserve physical health and beauty, allowing the individual more confidence in themselves.

Dr. Keith Kanner, Host/Anchor of Your Family Matters TV/Radio, Author of *Your Family Matters*, Licensed & Board Certified Clinical Psychologist & Psychoanalyst

Middle Age Beauty

Soulful Secrets From a Former Face
Model Living Botox Free in her Forties

Middle Age Beauty

Soulful Secrets From a Former Face
Model Living Botox Free in her Forties

Machel Shull

AYNI
BOOKS

Winchester, UK
Washington, USA

First published by Ayni Books, 2013
Ayni Books is an imprint of John Hunt Publishing Ltd., Laurel House, Station Approach,
Alresford, Hants, SO24 9JH, UK
office1@jhpbooks.net
www.johnhuntpublishing.com
www.ayni-books.com

For distributor details and how to order please visit the 'Ordering' section on our website.

Text copyright: Machel Shull 2013

ISBN: 978 1 78099 574 8

A CIP catalogue record for this book is available from the British Library.

Design: Stuart Davies

Printed and bound by CPI Group (UK) Ltd, Croydon, CR0 4YY

Medical disclaimer: This book is not intended as a substitute for the
medical advice of physicians. The reader should regularly consult a
physician in matters relating to his/her health and particularly with
respect to any symptoms that may require diagnosis or medical
attention. The author and the publisher specifically disclaim all
responsibility for any liability from any application of this book. If you
need advice or medical help, do consult your doctor.

We operate a distinctive and ethical publishing philosophy in all
areas of our business, from our global network of authors to
production and worldwide distribution.

CONTENTS

For my husband, Robin and my son, Jackson
AND
My parents Micky and William Penn

Acknowledgements

I would like to acknowledge John Hunt Publishing for seeing the potential and need for a positive book urging women to care more about their natural beauty and their soul. I would also like to recognize my son Jackson Tuck. He is an inspiration to me every day as his mother.

I would like to acknowledge Michiko Rolek, my first mentor, for giving me wings to fly. Thank you to Dr. Tess Hightower for reading my very first pages of another book and encouraging my love for writing. Thank you to Dr. Reiter, Dr. Patricia Bragg, Dr. Mike Moreno, Dr. Anthony F. Smith, Dr. Kim Kelly and Lauren Antonucci for allowing me to interview you all on how to enrich our lives and gain optimum health during our middle age beauty period. Thank you to my wonderful supportive husband, Robin Shull. Your love and support on this journey has given me more courage to write and reveal more because of your help. I would also like to thank someone no longer on this earth, my Grandma Lula. Thank you, Grandma, for helping me find early pearls of wisdom that would forever alter my journey. Sometimes just like in the movie credits, that last person mentioned is just as important as the first. Thank you to my mother, Micky Penn. Her support and encouraging insights helped me stay focused and on point so I could reach within to write *Middle Age Beauty*.

Foreword

It has been said that we are all students and teachers to each other. My students are my best teachers; together we explore what works and what doesn't on the inner journey of finding and loving ourselves. And Machel is one of those students that are a light in the world. Her book *Middle Age Beauty* is teaching us that being true to ourselves allows our beauty to shine through. She shares her beautiful honesty and reveals that true beauty is our integrity.

I am honored to be a part of Machel's path called *Middle Age Beauty*, restoring the soul through finding the true self. We both resonate with the illuminating words of Audrey Hepburn:

> *The beauty of a woman is not in a facial mode, but the true beauty in a woman is reflected in her soul. It is the caring that she lovingly gives, the passion that she shows. The beauty of a woman grows with the passing years.*

Machel gives us a true gem, filled with insightful tips and tools to capture more meaning, value and purpose in our everyday lives. She reminds me to age both exquisitely and gratefully at almost 56 with the ultimate secret, identify more with the soul's inner life, our humanity and practice of shifting from a worrier to warrior. Also by connecting to our spirit through meditation, we tap into our forever young spiritedness and have a reservoir of inexhaustible *zenergy*. I am inspired to take her *Friendship quiz* and make more time for Seinfeld like Moments. Because no matter what the age, 'girls just wanna have fun' or Fun-Zen, according to my fifteen year old daughter Grace. I am adding *Middle Age Beauty* to my selected few bedside books. With Machel's light to guide us home to our true beautiful selves, we can celebrate being the hero of our own story.

MJ Rolek, Author of *Mental Fitness, Complete Workouts for Body, Mind, and Soul*

A Woman does not become interesting until she is over forty.
~ Coco Chanel

Dear Readers,

Before I share with you why your soul is more important than a Botox injection at the plastic surgeon's office, I want you to know that I understand the quest for looking young. I am a woman that secretly dreaded becoming middle-aged, too. And why would I not with quotes like "A forty year old single woman is more likely to be killed by a terrorist than to ever marry."

You've heard the slang word 'cougar' comparing women to a four-legged animal because they are successfully dating a younger man. You've seen the reality shows depicting women as cat-fighting, angry, belligerent and indecent friends, while sipping their wine and smiling with their plump lips. You've seen those commercials telling women over the age of forty that their eyelashes are falling out. That they may feel lethargic and look exhausted so now is the time to buy a 'chin lift'. You've heard those rumors when female stars fall from their crescent heights because now they are no longer an ingénue.

You've watched every rerun of Sex and the City. You know the names of four single characters. You've watched these women discuss every weekend over brunch the logistics of moving through their midlife with cunning precision. Almost as if these fictional women lived in a war zone in New York City because they are older, single women clinging on to their friendships and moments passed...

What can I tell you? I hit upon a mild depression the month of my fortieth birthday. Maybe all of those factors mentioned above had subconsciously preyed on my own insecurities about my age. I felt like such a cliché that week. I had called my mom on the phone to explain to her that I had no idea why I felt queasy regarding turning one year older. I had a heaviness that just sat on my chest. I felt paralyzed about my age. I didn't want to 'feel expired'. I know from discussing with others now this experience I had can be common. Though many of us keep it 'hush-hush'.

Now I must let you in on the biggest shock of my life. Guess what happened when I turned forty? I woke up happy! Life continued. I ended up having the best year ever. My health, beauty and attitude felt like they were in sync for the first time. I had this grounded feeling of getting to a destination I had always heard about, and wondered, "Is this it? What's the big fuss anyway? The view is wonderful from here!"

To arrive at this moment was not easy. As a former model that felt expired at the age of twenty, and an actress that felt semi-expired at the age of thirty, you can only imagine what I truly thought of that midlife period.

Now I am on the other side looking back at all of my expiration dates. Why had I allowed myself to buy into a viewpoint which was not based on my own path? After much reflection, I realized that after twenty years of trying to walk a fine line based on beauty and age, I have uncovered secrets that can help you feel more radiant with each passing year. From working with a Zen Master Life Coach to being a face model in Los Angeles, this diverse background has lead to my own personal discovery of what I call the Beauty Trinity. In the midst of these three sections, I will also share some of my own personal struggles that lead me to discover a more meaningful, mindful existence during the second half of my life.

You don't need to buy into the 'expiration date dilemma'. While plastic surgery ads to even your own peer group might have you believe your time is up because of your age, this book is embracing soulful choices and simple beauty tips that embrace... guess what?

The Real You.

Thank you for taking this journey with me.

~ Machel Shull

Introduction

When I was fifteen my parents enrolled me in a modeling class because I did not make the volleyball team when I was a sophomore in high school. I had played volleyball for four years prior. But when the new coach came to town, I just didn't have the serve I needed. If you know anything about high school, this was quite a traumatic loss. Little did I know this fork in the road would set my life on a different path.

While my girlfriends were hanging with their cliques and doing cheerleading splits, I was driving to Kansas City to work as a model for Hallmark. Instead of spending hours in tanning beds, I avoided wearing shorts because of my ghastly white legs. Instead of wearing heavy layers of makeup, I learned how to apply my makeup with a more natural approach. These moments laid the foundation for the next fifteen years of taking care of my health and beauty as a model and an actress.

I have learned important fashion choices, health and beauty tips because of growing up as a model in this competitive field. Learning inside secrets as a model, I still carry them with me today as a 41 year old woman. These are secrets some would tell you won't work. They are inside tips that might even shock you. Those that would have you believe they don't work are the plastic surgeons, the medical spas and those that want you to believe that being natural is *out*. Saving your money and feeling great about your soul, health and looks are definitely *in*.

This book is about embracing your natural you. *Middle Age Beauty* is a quest in finding a deeper connection to your soul, while focusing on how to optimize your health and feel beautiful in your *own* skin.

I will point out some inexpensive beauty secrets that you might have missed if you weren't a model or had a close friend that knew these tricks. In my Health section I will give you some important suggestions that have improved my overall sense of well-being. This also includes one smart diet choice that has been profiled on Dr. Phil and the show *The Doctors*. This diet is more like a 'lifestyle' than just a fad. This book will help you set important standards in your daily routine that can help you discover more soulful, mindful moments with yourself and your friends.

First I share with you the 'Three Dos'. This will reveal one *lie* that must be stopped, one *face* that needs protecting, and one *joy* that carries the secret to your daily happiness.

Part One will tackle the absolute most important part of this book. Your soul. Are you nurturing the inner you? Your soul is the most important part of this equation of the beauty trinity. I will share with you simple steps that can help you feel more relaxed, connected and inspired by taking some powerful steps to examine your social life, and how you spend your time. I will also share with you what famous movie fighter should inspire you to climb the steps to your own dreams.

Part Two will be a comprehensive look into how to stay healthy easily, while embracing smart diets that DO work. Also, you might be horrified when I tell you the one absolute thing you have to give up if you want to stay and look younger *longer*. It's a matter of sophistication versus health. Part Three will break down the products that you can buy today under $20.00. I will explain to you with my background with beauty products as a model why these certain tricks work.

These three parts SOUL, HEALTH and BEAUTY form the important beauty trinity that determines our feeling of self-worth, feeling ageless and ignoring the pressure to add toxins to our body just to beat out a wrinkle.

I am excited to also share with you interviews from top experts in the field of Health, Beauty and Psychology that reveal important factors you need to know in your quest in developing your own beauty equation:

Dr. Patricia Bragg – the daughter of the first health crusader in America. She is also a doctor, motivational speaking coach, author and business entrepreneur.

MJ Rolek – is the great-granddaughter to the first Zen Master to make his home in America. She is also an author and Zen life meditation coach in Los Angeles.

Dr. Mike Moreno – *New York Times* Bestselling Author of *The 17 Day Diet* reveals key steps in staying healthy.

Dr. Tess Hightower – A psychiatrist and author from Beverly Hills that has been featured on many television shows for her field of expertise on relationships. She will uncover why women shouldn't ever lie about their age.

Dr. Russel J. Reiter – An insightful interview with a doctor and teacher in medical neuroscience that reveals a key hormone which fights aging naturally.

New York Health Expert Lauren Antonucci – A nutritionist and Health Expert that helps guide patients every day to make healthier choices with their lives.

Dr. Kim Kelly – A Southern Californian Homeopathic Doctor that reveals the one needle that is okay to inject into your skin for beneficial health reasons.

Dr. Anthony F. Smith – Co-founder and Managing Director of Leadership Research Institute, Bestselling Author and Professor of Leadership shares an insightful interview on why women have excellent leadership skills. Plus, why women are natural born leaders in and out of the work force.

An American Poet Louise Bogan so accurately described in one of her poems the conundrum we women face in the Millennium:

I cannot believe that the inscrutable universe turns on an axis of suffering; surely the strange beauty of the world must somewhere rest on pure joy!

To label women anything but beautiful for just making it gracefully to this place in our lives, remember that quote.

Remember that this world is ours to take back. Our beauty is in our own integrity as we embrace our middle-aged years with a new sense of wonder and excitement. Join me on this journey to finding soulful secrets, feeling healthy and looking younger naturally with *your* own dignity and grace.

The 3 Dos

I always wanted to be somebody, but now I realize I should have been more specific.

~ Lily Tomlin

Chapter 1

Do Tell the Truth about Your Age. After All, It's Only a Number

I went to a party at the beginning of the holidays last year in The Crosby, which just happens to be a gated community with many wealthy residents. This is not an important factor. I am just trying set the scene for you. Marble floors, opulent chandeliers, tight dresses, stiletto heels and yuletide greetings buzzing around me as I entered onto the scene.

You see, I write a column in a newspaper covering social gatherings. So I am often invited to the lavish parties in the Rancho Santa Fe community. I tend to mingle in and out of this world like bubbles flow inside champagne… naturally. When one of the lovely mature ladies approached me for conversation, I welcomed her into my space. We then began our small talk quite innocently.

"You look lovely tonight, Machel," Ellen said to me. (Not her real name.)

"Thanks, Ellen. So do you." And, she did. Ellen was a beautiful woman with a slender build and elegant face that put you in mind of Zsa Zsa Gabor.

"Your skin looks amazing."

"You are too sweet," I reply. My skin tends to be my strong suit with my looks. I am not stick thin with fake boobs. But luckily great genetics and a few of my own tricks have kept my skin looking younger than my actual age.

"What do you do?" Ellen asks

"What do you mean?" I ask coyly.

"What have you had done?" Ellen asks.

"Honestly, I haven't done anything to my face. I have some wives' tale-like tricks that work. I keep it simple, you could say."

"Well whatever you are doing it's working, honey."

"Thanks, Ellen." She is being genuine and I have always liked Ellen. "I appreciate the compliment. I am now 41 and I feel good about being natural."

"Oh, Honey, never, never tell anyone how old you are. It's just not necessary," she says with her pretty red lips puckered with a patronizing tone. I don't think that she meant to be rude. Ellen was just trying to educate me on the 'world to come' as an older woman.

That's when I said it. It just flew out of my mouth. I didn't mean to sound so indignant but I think I did slightly, and felt very proud of my response to her. "Ellen, I didn't make it this far to keep my age a secret. I worked too hard to look great to now keep it a secret. Who cares what anyone else thinks." Wow, did you hear that? That remark felt like leaps and bounds for me after crawling past the big four-zero.

With all of the Latisse commercials about how tired we look in our forties you can't really blame Ellen for trying to educate me on the 'point of view' the world has on aging. I have made an active stance on my age. If someone asks, I tell. I don't round off the number or say with a glib expression, "I'm holding at 39." I just knock them dead with the truth. You should try it, too. Telling the truth about your age is liberating. There is something about just being so honest, that most are shocked with your honest response.

The number one 'Do' is to be honest about your age. If you are one of those women that conceal or lie about your age, stop and ask yourself why you are doing it? Isn't it a rather terrible exception we allow as an *okay* thing to lie about? I know that you can't blame women for maybe fibbing just a little now and then.

Society, friends and peer groups can be downright cruel. As I have learned from my own personal experience, I, too have been taught that I will expire with age. Why with that destructive thought in our heads, why would we not consider at least making allowances for this one little lie?

This is where we – I mean women as a collective whole – need to work together to change this thought. I say we stop this nonsense now. This is no way to train our children, our daughters and our sons or future generations because we have allowed ourselves to be bullied into feeling like our age might make us seem less attractive or subtract from our self-worth. (If you are honestly telling the truth about your age and over the age of forty you can skip ahead to the next 'Do'. This chapter does not apply to you.)

After the party was over, I went home and slipped into my comfortable flannel pink pajamas. Then I turned on my computer to do some important research. Well, not really like extensive or anything causing me to lose sleep at night; I'm talking like Facebook. I researched my group of peers and noticed a current trend for most women: they hide the year they were born. The month and the day were posted. The year, however, was missing. Then I remembered to check my own profile. Was I guilty, too? And, there it was: February 22, _____ without the year I was born. I quickly changed it. I would no longer be one of those women that remained ageless because I was afraid of a number defining my age.

After that opulent evening of hanging out with the socialites in Rancho Santa Fe, I turned the corner on my own insecurity regarding my age. I actually listed my actual FULL birthday on Facebook. I know. This is not a massive triumph in life. However, just like the author Gregg Braden searching for a better outcome for the Millennium in *The Isaiah Effect*, I am on a mission to try and reverse women's thinking on why we need to care more about being true to ourselves and worry less about a greedy society that would have us looking like plastic dolls with fake lips.

After this experience, I wanted to dig down deeper and find out from an expert their thoughts on exactly how this one little lie for women can cause irrevocable damage in the long-term for ourselves. So I reached into my roster of phone numbers the next day. I sat and pondered who could I call to find out more answers on what this one little lie can do to a woman's self-esteem. Then I knew whom I would call. Dr. Tess Hightower, my psychiatrist, from my twenties decade.

Well, I know what you might be thinking. This isn't something I ever thought I would brag about. However, I take great pride in 'my younger self' being wise enough to seek counsel when I needed it the most. You see, just like many actresses in Hollywood, I had an acting coach. John Kirby was kind enough to make my introduction to Tess Hightower when I needed some counseling during a pivotal point during my twenties.

On a side note, I must tell you that studying acting is one of the most important gifts that came out of my modeling days. Acting is essentially about studying a character that you are working on for a part, a play, or for a movie. In order to play this part you must know who the character is, which means exploration of your imagination and emotions. Instead of being frightened of my feelings or wanting to numb them with medication, I have always embraced my highs and lows. Acting classes encouraged exploration of feelings, which helped me become more 'in tune' with myself. So when John Kirby told me, "You must see my good friend Tess, I think you will like her," I listened.

Originally growing up on a farm in Missouri in the Ozark Mountains, do think Elly May Clampett from *The Beverly Hillbillies* here on my part. At this stage in the game I had not become familiar with and did not accept therapy as being 'normal'. I thought I must be crazy if I went to see a doctor regarding my psyche. Since John Kirby was a man I trusted, I grew and matured immensely when I took his advice. I swallowed my fears, gathered my thoughts and walked right up to her doorstep and into her office.

When I met Tess at first I was shocked. First of all, Tess is beautiful. Do imagine a Grace Kelly type wearing glasses, and elegant, tailored clothes. Dr. Tess was the most grounded and surreal woman I had ever met at this point in my life. Her encouragement of looking within and exploring my fears helped me see how some of my own limited thinking had actually caused my sudden feelings of loss. Although beauty is skin deep, there is no miracle cure in making you feel better about yourself if you are not content on the inside with what is going on in your soul. This part is relevant because meeting Dr. Tess helped me in my footing on my path to Middle Age Beauty.

I met with Dr. Tess off and on over the years for support and guidance, which gave me much insight regarding myself and my relationships to those around me. I managed to work through some of my own insecurities, rebuild my thinking and discover a young girl that still had an idea of what I wanted my life to represent, and how I could make important strides by taking action and real steps to become the woman I always wanted to be.

Life moves forward, years pass but some connections always remain. When I contacted Dr. Tess regarding my search on 'Lying about the age bit' she had her own stories to share with me that reinforced my idea that women should begin a new movement and preach to the mountaintops about their real age like in the days of burning bras, and forgetting those apron days and making stacks of pancakes during the decade of the fifties. I had to dig deeper for answers from someone that knows more about *why* it's important to be honest about our age *always*.

Here is my interview with Dr. Tess Hightower regarding the ramifications of lying about your age:

What side effects do you think can happen to a woman's psyche when she lies about her age to others?

Dr. Tess: When women lie to others about their age, what they don't realize is that they are basically lying to themselves. Living in Los Angeles (Beverly Hills) for 62 years, I've seen this so many times. There is such pressure from society not to age. I've even been to funerals where they had an open casket and noticed that this poor deceased person is made-up and dressed up as if they weren't dead. A beautiful woman dies two deaths... once and when they lose their beauty.

As a psychologist and authority on mental health, do you see a strong correlation with mental health and aging? If one does not seek to learn about their inner self and dynamics of their character – do you feel ultimately an unsound mind can contribute to you aging?

Dr. Tess: For the most part, I find that when men and women are fully engaged in life, doing something they are passionate about, or something that gives their lives meaning, I find that these people are less concerned with the aging process – they are just busy living their lives. All of the above takes care of the inner dynamics – but if all you have to offer is the external – well when that begins to fade, you are in trouble. And yes, if you continually obsess about how you look rather than who you are as a person, it can contribute to mental pathologies.

Do you feel that aging can be related to unhappiness?

Dr. Tess: Of course! For all of the reasons listed above. If all you feel you have to offer is how beautiful you are... well someone will always come along who is prettier, taller, thinner, tanner and, well as we age, younger! If you are 50 trying to look 30 – my guess is that you will pretty much make yourself unhappy. Stepping outside of yourself and being there for others (such as volunteering) can take years off of your life – that good feeling just oozes out!

Do you feel reaching middle age in your life is actually a wonderful age to be and why?

Dr. Tess: Absolutely! I will be 64 this summer and not so unhappy when I look in the mirror. The best years of my life were my fifties. I never felt more comfortable in my skin, more sure of my career and of knowing who I am in the world. Oh sure, I have a few more wrinkles and a few more pounds – but my husband tells me I am beautiful! So maybe finding the right partner is part of the key!

Do you have any stories that relate to you personally regarding aging that might be insightful for others?

Dr. Tess: A few years ago, maybe when I was 55 – I had one of those dreaded health check-ups you endure at a certain age in life. I had to be there very early in the morning, I think around 6:00am. So I arrive, in sweats, ponytail on the top of my head, sans makeup of course. The anesthesiologist comes up and begins asking me important medical questions. He then looks at me and says – "You look pretty good, Tess, for 55 – have you had work done?" I'm already grumpy for having to be up so early and have THIS test. I glare at him and say, "No, so far I haven't had the need to cut off half my face and throw it into the trash bin." He began to laugh hysterically, and said, "Oh my God, I love it, I have to go and phone my wife and tell her."

After connecting with Tess, the one quote that sent a shiver down my spine was: *"A beautiful woman dies two deaths, once and when they lose their beauty."* If this can be true, the most important factor for us in our Middle Age Beauty time is to find meaning and depth to our connections and our purpose here. If beauty will not last forever, maybe there is an important factor of learning to allow our natural beauty to be what it is and *do* age gracefully. We need to look deeper. Seeking approval from one's self also can alleviate the need to feel validated from a society that may never give us the spotlight and the glamour we were expecting as we grew older.

We don't want to end up like the character Norma Desmond in the infamous Hollywood movie, *Sunset Boulevard*. Do you remember that eerie ending as Norma, played by Gloria

Swanson, descended down the staircase declaring, "I'm ready for my close-up."? Unfortunately, life can imitate fiction and the lights can dim on us without warning.

When a moment like that can descend on your thoughts and prey on your own insecurities, remind yourself of this fact. Being your age is actually a miracle. Not everyone makes it to this stage. Sometimes accidents happen. Disease or disaster strikes. Each added day is a blessing. So why not learn to count our age as that – *a blessing.*

Women, are you ready to start the movement? Are you ready to put behind you those years of concealing and lying about who you are and where you are in your journey? Take the leap of faith. Dare to break the mold. Stand proud and admit your age... even to yourself. Remember *do* tell the truth about your age. After all, it's *only* a number.

Chapter 2

Do Say Yes To Your Natural Self. After All, There is Only ONE of You

We sat outside eating leafy green salads under the eucalyptus trees. Five women dressed in designer wear from head to toe enjoyed the perfect sunny weather on the terrace at the fancy inn located in the heart of one of Southern California's desired zip codes.

Each woman wore their own form of sunblock: A hat, SPF 70 by Neutrogena, Oil of Olay 15 Daily lotion or just heavy anti-aging cover-up makeup that shielded their skin during the lunch hour. The conversation ranged from designer purses, husbands, children's accolades, to last but not least... *Botox*.

That's usually when I turn to glance at the trees in a casual manner. Almost as if I am in deep thought like I am studying the roots of the eucalyptus trees and trying to determine why they grow so close to the surface here in Rancho Santa Fe. Could there be a correlation? Then I check my purse to make sure no one can see my one dollar anti-aging secret I always carry in my purse, which isn't Louis Vuitton or Prada. Think more along the lines of Kenneth Cole, Franco Sarto. I can find these brands at the budget stores and feel almost decent enough to sit under the sun with the rest of my friends displaying Gucci and Prada bags.

They never ask me. You know, about the Botox thing. This is when I become the invisible one. My girlfriends know that I do not use it. Sometimes I'll quip just to sound like part of the conversation so I can fit in to the air surrounding me in my tightly-knit support group of friends: "I know, I may need it and will definitely use some in the future." Meanwhile, I know that this is not true. I am falling prey to wanting to feel the seal of approval of the Botox clique that can be found in almost any town in America.

That is when I check my handbag to make sure my secret is not exposed. My secret doesn't sound as glamorous as Botox. You might think it's even ridiculous when you find out. I don't. Why? Because it works. I will reveal in Part Three my *one dollar secret* that even makes it through the tight airport security checks and will not be confiscated from you before you board your flight to your amazing destination. No kidding. I will devote one entire chapter to this subject later. For now let's return back to the five women and their leafy green salads.

The conversation drifts from Kim Kardashian to why adding layers to your body can make you look fat when you should always try and look thin.

I enjoyed our surroundings under the bright blue sky, taking in the frivolousness of our conversation. Sometimes it's nice to be distracted, relax and think of the prettier things that can give us temporary satisfaction. You know, that quick fix like that right designer lipstick or perfect pedicure nail color that you would only reveal to your inner circle because you don't mind sharing beauty secrets.

But is Botox really a beauty secret? Is a needle injection to the face just so accepted now that there is no cause for caution or investigating?

Let's get down to the 'nitty-gritty' as they say.

Okay, okay, plastic surgery? Well, yes, there is a reconstructive need. And, yes, if there is *truly* a need. But mini facelifts, lip injections, and face fillers? Do you really know what you are putting into your face? What are the long-term effects? If Botox was just approved in 2003, where are the examples for us to see of what someone will look like in twenty years? How can we measure the real significance of what using Botox can do to your face?

So maybe you only have it once in a year. All I am suggesting is to investigate the facts before you fill your *only face* with a substance that is known to make your muscles atrophy when abused over and over.

Here are some up close and personal facts you may want to consider before you seek a needle to help hide a wrinkle temporarily. (Botox wears off and only lasts for a few months. Those of you Botox lovers that obviously know this, keep reading just in case you haven't heard or read some of the recent studies that reveal a darker side to this quick fix wrinkle fix.)

According to much extensive research online, there are some disturbing facts you might have missed from your local medical spa doctor or the countless ads women and men are subjected to on a daily basis on the Internet. I'm not even mentioning the ads in fashion magazines, television, or just the peer pressure you may feel like I did in the story I outlined at lunchtime with my group of friends. My own personal daily experience with this *toxin* that has gained acceptance, notoriety and is now even used by women in their twenties! The popular filler can be found at a Botox Party. Where this toxin is passed around like a pastry to their guests.

"Why, yes, I would like an injection, please."

The waitress passes the needle.

This is not an exaggeration. If you live on the west coast of the United States or in any metropolis area anywhere in the world, you have heard about them, or had a friend that attended one of these gatherings.

You might be thinking, "If they are doing it why shouldn't I at least try Botox, too?"

Well, you already know that I am taking the approach to aging natural here. I am asking you, too, to take a more direct look before you decide to add a foreign toxin into your bloodstream. Find out what you could be risking all for the sake of trying to make a line if you will dissolve beneath the skin.

I have one word. It is enough for me: Poison. The mere fact that Botox is from Botulism is enough to keep this forty-something woman adding her dollar creams with secret delight as my own resourceful measures toward anti-aging, without spending too much money just to sound trendy and to fit in at a luncheon.

Here are the facts on Botox:

- Botulinum toxin is the true name for Botox. Just like cigarettes were once used for asthma, look for future changes with medical warnings to be issued as time keeps on giving us more time to research this new trendy, cool poison.
- In 2008, the FDA announced that Botox had been the source for "adverse reactions, sometimes including respiratory failure and death."
- In 2009, the Canadian Government issued a warning to their residents regarding the use of Botox. If using this as an injection for any kind of treatment, including for anti-aging, an adverse reaction can occur to other parts of your body. This can cause muscle atrophy, pneumonia, breathing and speech disorders.
- In June 2011, *The New York Times* covered a story based on one by David T. Neal and Tanya L. Chartrand, published in *Social Psychological and Personality Science* that Botox can actually lesson someone's ability to feel or to feel empathy.
- According to world famous nutritionist and author Dr. Nicholas Perricone, Botox paralyzes our face muscles, which eventually can inadvertently add to signs of aging. The opposite effect of what you want.

Before Botox ask yourself these few questions:

- What other methods can I use before filling my ONLY face with a poison?
- Has there been enough history behind Botox to even inject it into my skin?

- Would my grandmother be okay with me using Botox?
- Will Botox just stay in the area in my skin where it was injected or will it travel to other parts of my body? What kind of damage can it do if that happens?
- Is a wrinkle worth compromising my health over?
- Is it possible this treatment will cause me to age faster than aging just naturally?

The bottom line is simply this: Your face is the *only* one you have. Don't just buy into the peer pressure of trying to stay younger looking by following suit after famous folks that glamorize this on television. If you have had some Botox... don't use it anymore! Do your own research first. Sophia Loren had this to say about natural beauty: *"Beauty is how you feel inside and it reflects in your eyes. It is not something physical."* So remember there is only *one* you in this world. Embrace your natural beauty. Find other ways to keep wrinkles away that don't require injecting a needle into your face.

Chapter 3

Do One Act a Day for Yourself that Brings You Inner Joy –
After All, YOU are Important

Sitting inside the parking lot at the pharmacy over twelve years ago, I managed to feed my crying baby in the back seat of my black Ford Expedition. I had just moved down from Los Angeles to the San Diego area. Not only did I not know anyone, I had just lost a familiar world of living in Los Angeles with all of my friends, daily routines and the days when all I did was think of myself, my wants and my needs.

Motherhood changed all of that for me. Being my son's mother brought a foundation of stability within me and also helped shed some light on a few necessities in life… like keeping a newborn alive. That was honestly what consumed me at that moment in time. Everyone knows that babies are blessings. Everyone knows that motherhood can be trying. But until you actually become a mother for the first time, you really cannot know what those harried moments feel like until you are sitting with a screaming baby alone in a parking lot, afraid to move.

Which brings me back to that moment in the parking lot. I had felt completely overwhelmed, out of place in suburbia and just exhausted.

I woke up with one thought every day: "I must keep the baby alive!" I drove around with my baby in his car seat in tow trying to shake off the raw nerves of motherhood, while listening to the Goo Goo Dolls.

Well, at least I did not have one of those stickers on my car that said "Baby on Board", but I might as well have. As I sat in the back seat next to my inconsolable baby, I felt invisible to the world. I watched another mother with her son walk into the pharmacy with a bright smile. Arm and arm, son and mom walked like life was easy and they were right where they should be. How would I ever get to that moment? I wondered.

That was when it hit me. I was having one of those self-pitying moments where time stops and the world feels bleak. I was truly one of those mothers that strived too hard for perfection...which we all know does not exist in life. Somewhere between the loss of sleep, losing friends and moving to a new environment I had forgotten to just relax a bit... plus make some time for someone very important:

Me

My life then consisted of cooking and baby time. I made pot roasts, salmon dinners and perfect sunny-side eggs with two crisp pieces of bacon next to two sliced tomatoes every morning for my husband. I brought him breakfast every day on a tray. I brought in the paper. I made the coffee. I changed the diapers. I read children's books to my baby hoping he would understand and become one of those Mozart babies with a high IQ. I tucked him in every night. I stood over his crib and watched him to make sure he never stopped breathing.

Motherhood and my new life was... *exhausting and beautiful, too.*

I only had two goals at that time in my life: *Be a good wife and mother.* I wrote them out on a piece of paper inside a journal. These two words defined what I was then. Of course, I would not realize until that moment in the back seat at the parking lot with my baby that there was something significantly missing in this picture:

A goal that included a desire for myself.

Although both of my goals were admirable, they were both selfless, too. There was not a stitch of what brought my soul inner joy anywhere in this equation... that day when I realized this, I began to cry, too. There I was sobbing in the back of my shiny black SUV right next to my crying baby.

Luckily, the back windows were tinted black so I don't think that too many witnessed this moment of pity. You know, the new town, and the new quietness of motherhood hours would just stretch out endlessly. I remember thinking, "How in the world can I make these 24 hours pass?" I didn't know honestly. I thought my moments of fun were up.

I am sharing with you this inside story so you know that during this particular time I forgot one important factor. I forgot to make *myself* a priority, too. All of the small things that had given me joy were set aside because I had not 'included my needs' as an important goal.

This was probably one of the more challenging periods in my life. Do you tend to make others your first priority and forget to make yourself happy, too? If so, it's easy to forget the small joys that can bring us hope. One of my favorite quotes delves into this topic perfectly. *"Many people lose the small joys in the hope for the big happiness."* Author and Nobel Prize winner Pearl S. Buck captures in that quote the essence of this chapter. Sometimes we can lose much happiness in the midst of our lives aiming for something too perfect or what we think will bring us happiness.

My story about being a mother is my best example to you on how I learned to never stop forgetting about my needs, too. You don't need to be a mother to neglect yourself. Life can feel like a constant struggle of things to do and places to see, that leaves us little time to enjoy moments of bliss.

That's why the number three 'Do' is do one thing a day that brings you inner joy. So the question is, do you know what small things bring you a sense of peace? If you don't, do take this time to think about that statement. Stop reading, and write out at least three things that make you happy.

Now I am not referring to something like winning the lottery. I'm not talking about spending money like some vacuous shopper or buying your favorite pair of Manolos. I am talking about *a simple act* that can fit into your daily schedule. Here is my list that I choose from throughout my busy week of work, writing deadlines, motherhood, marketing and helping my husband run his business. Life is busy for all of us! It is up to us to make time for an inner joy that will make this one day in our life just a little brighter because we happened to remember someone very special:

Yourself.

My List:

Drink coffee in the morning.

Feed the birds in my backyard.

Go for a fifteen-minute walk in the neighborhood.

Make time to read a book.

Go to a juice shop and buy a smoothie that tastes delicious.

Buy an Americana, which is an espresso with water at a coffee shop.

Call my mom.

Call my sister or girlfriends to chat.

Go for a run.

Visit my favorite bookstore and buy a new novel to read.

You see, these are all obtainable, specific tasks that don't require much money. These are simple things that I know make me feel moments of bliss during my daily routine. The trick is to *schedule* them in so you don't miss it!

Often on our journey at different periods and chapters it will be challenging to make time for what can bring us moments of inner joy. However, if we forget to nourish our soul along the way, our lives can feel out-of-sorts and lack a deeper meaning.

As you see my list has nothing to do with my family because I devote my time and energy to them daily. These are simple tasks that I know make my world just a bit brighter, bringing less stress and more love to help nourish my inner soul that still needs to feel loved. This point makes it in the prequel because I find most of us forget to take time for our own desires.

Ultimately, by taking care of yourself and experiencing small moments of joy, you awaken and connect to your soul. You must take time to build up your spirit each day so that smile you wish to find can happen naturally. As one of my favorite philosophers Norman Vincent Peale often said, *"Say Yes to Life!"* He encouraged adding these three words to the beginning of your day in one of my favorite books, the *Treasury of Joy and Enthusiasm*:

Just for today I will be happy, I will take care of my body, I will try to strengthen my mind, I will exercise my soul in three ways, I will be agreeable, I will have a program...

This book by the late Norman Vincent Peale is withered and worn on my bedside table. However, this book still holds some valuable suggestions that have helped and encouraged me during difficult and challenging times. So remember that You are the most important part of your equation. Your attitude, your spirit count toward the Middle Age Beauty equation. So make time for just ONE thing that will bring you inner joy each day.

If you are wondering, I did manage to leave the parking lot that day. My son also stopped crying. That day just happened to be the day I made a U-turn and went back to the Jamba Juice right next to the pharmacy. My son quietly enjoyed his binky while we stood in line. I remember listening to the humming of the blenders, enjoying the smell of the fresh fruit and feeling excited to take one moment for me. That day, I remembered someone important to my son that mattered: His mother. *Remember, after all, you count! Life is yours for the taking.*

Part One – Your Soul

We all live in suspense from day to day, from hour to hour; in other words, we are the hero of our own story.
~ American Author, Mary McCarthy

Chapter 4

Important Questions for the Soul

In 1997, I met a beautiful woman, named Michiko Rolek. Of Japanese descent from the first Zen master to ever make his home in America, imagine an oval face of wisdom with the sweetest eyes that look like the 'all knowing to the soul'. I stood in line waiting to pick up my coffee marked 'Michelle', the wrong name, which happens to be a common theme in my life since my name is unusual.

The air in the tightly air-conditioned Starbucks near Warner Brothers studio in the Valley in Los Angeles was packed with the usual artsy type reading and writing on top of oval tables, while this woman I was about to meet sat perfectly upright with perfect posture looking like a sparkling ballerina on point waiting patiently for me to join her. What I did not know is I was about to meet the person that would become one of the most positive influences of my life. Michiko Rolek had just had her book published, *Mental Fitness, Complete Workouts for the Body, Mind, and Soul*. I had not read her book. And honestly I did not know anything about Michiko except that she might be able to help me calm my nerves before I auditioned as an actress. I had hit upon a stumbling block in Hollywood.

I had lost my confidence after a few solid years of booking commercial and television appearances; one day, it was like I woke up and suddenly was afraid and didn't know what I was afraid of... you know, just like 'the mean reds' in *Breakfast at Tiffany's*. Well, I was still searching for a place with deeper roots, a place that connected me to my *soul*. Now this isn't about religion. This is about digging within to the innermost part of your quiet self and reaching for meaning and sure footing. Somehow I had lost mine after seven years in the acting business.

Finally, I took my seat across from Michiko with my coffee. I believe she was wearing a pink cool zipper jacket with jewels. I fumbled with my notepad (I always tried to come like I was prepared!) slightly intimidated by her intense, honest eye contact.

Okay, let me be honest. I was a mess. I felt vulnerable. I was freaked out. I had hit my mid-twenties and started to doubt almost every move I made in the commercial acting business. If you know anything about Hollywood, this type of energy can kill any audition and your career. At least I had been smart enough to ask for some much needed help. I had enrolled in an acting class per my Beverly Hills' agents' advice and I did not mesh with the acting teacher or her method of teaching. (I am filling you in on this because this is ultimately what brought me to the Starbucks.) After studying for one month in this class, I literally felt like a raw open wound, unable and too afraid to set foot out of my guesthouse in Studio City. Each week this teacher would have us scream for one minute straight, then laugh for the next, cry, yell and purge every emotion your body had in you into a room, with 35 other screaming acting students that actually looked like they knew what they were doing. I felt confused and dazed. I remember looking around wondering, "Am I missing something here?" Then I would think, "Is this why I am in Los Angeles, to do this?" Needless to say it wasn't. I had been a model first and my agents propelled me into commercials, then to acting auditions and so on. My career shifted so fast into the other, I never had a chance to question if that's what I truly wanted with my life's direction.

Michiko was kind enough that day to talk first because she could recognize that I could not. I listened to her speak quiet words of positivity that felt like an army of angels lifting me up and away from my chaotic thinking.

At the Starbucks that day I went over all of this with Michiko. I explained to her my inner struggle to find my footing. I wanted to know the meaning of why I was there, and if acting was what I should still be doing. She took my hand and said something like, "Girl, we are going to find that."

Next thing you know I am working on learning how to meditate weekly at Michiko's house. Each week I would sit across from her and calmly meditate on the 'Why' quest I was on, and then stopped trying to figure that out, and calmed my mind and my nerves. She uncovered secrets to me that I did not know. Like how to go deeper and rest my mind and focus on my breath. Week by week, I found myself holding my head high again. I practiced my exercises of connecting to my breath. I looked forward to seeing this amazing woman. I felt like she was sharing the secrets of the universe with me.

In the book, *Course of Miracles*, there is a simple theory that: "*A miracle is a shift in perception.*" That is exactly what was beginning to happen to me. I found out that who I was did not belong in that strange acting class that had me writhing on the floor to be in touch with my emotions. I called my agents and let them know I would be switching teachers. There was a slight pause on the phone. My agent was not thrilled. Yet, to my surprise he listened to me. I broke free of a radical crazy acting class that honestly just didn't work for my personality.

Life continued on for me. My course, my chapters and, yes, Michiko remained. While she continued to do book signings and receive endorsements for her book, I kept working with her over the years during trying times to remember that my mind is only in essence thoughts that I can change when I have the courage to go deeper and face my own fears.

In this book, '*nourishing your soul*' is the most important truth of your ticket to finding real beauty. If you work on yourself, face your fears and are willing to see what your own weaknesses are, you can grow into the person you've always wanted to become. And it's never too late to start over and become who you really always wanted to be.

Luckily for me, the stars aligned when I found Michiko Rolek that day at the Starbucks. Since then Michiko has mentored many others, including stars, authors and just normal folks like me that needed a helping hand in the right direction. This part of the book will give you some light suggestions that are simple tips that can improve upon your current view on your path to finding a balance between beauty/soul/health.

Here is my interview with Life and Zen Coach Michiko Rolek:
In your book you describe "Mental Fitness" as about keeping your head strong and your mind clear. What small steps can we do to achieve a more centered state?
Michiko: Here are three small heart steps that will help you come home to yourself, your magical journey to center:

- Take deep slow breaths to and from your core. Engage your spiritual muscle, the diaphragm, to make sure the breaths are more effective. Tip: Taking soul time for three deep slow centering breaths during your daily rounds dissolves tension and brings you the comfort and joy of a clear mind and peaceful heart.
- Become posture aware, so you're upright instead of uptight. Upright posture keeps you too blessed to be stressed with a long back and strong core to weather any storm.
- Cultivate a daily ritual to practice counting your daisy chain of blessings. Gratitude gifts us with reflection, renewal and restores our perspective and sense of humor.

You have received many endorsements for your book, *Mental Fitness*, from heavy hitters like author and publisher Louise L. Hay and the author of *Don't Sweat the Small Stuff*, by Richard Carlson. You also are a descendant of Sokei-an Sasaki, the first Zen Master to make his home in America. What overall

message do you wish to share with women and men in the middle age beauty period experiencing fear regarding their age? What simple techniques can someone do to flush out these negative thoughts?

Michiko: The premise of my techniques, tools and tips is to honor Einstein's wise words which are rooted in Zen wisdom: "Out of clutter, find simplicity." The truth for me regarding fear and the middle age beauty period is about perception and seeing with new eyes. Other cultures and wisdom traditions respect the aging process, seeing getting older as a celebration of agelessness. I wholeheartedly agree and choose to age both gracefully and gratefully. The secret dancer's posture friendly tool, that I learned from my 'forever young' spirited 90 years of age mentor/author Auntie Helen Fleder is "The Miracle Diamond". Wearing the miracle diamond keeps us elongated or upright as mentioned. Consider, when we are aligned, we feel centered, stretched and strong, and negativity or the years cannot touch us. As Norman Vincent Peale once said, "Live your life, and forget your age." The Miracle Diamond motto: When the body lifts, the mind shifts, and the spirit soars.

As a Life Coach in Los Angeles, you have coached many famous stars in helping to achieve a more peaceful balance in their lives. You teach posture and breathing and relaxing techniques in *Mental Fitness*. I know from working with you personally that it is possible to learn these exercises and use them daily. How important is it to nourish our soul on a daily basis?

Michiko: The importance of nurturing our soul comes down to the choice of living a life of authenticity or quiet desperation. Bestselling author Sarah Ban Breathnach of *Simple Abundance* has impeccably said, "The authentic self is the soul made visible." Every breath, every step towards wholeness begins with the acceptance of the fact that you already possess the inner wisdom, the light of your soul to live your dreams. Tip: Food for your

Soul: Read more, Pray or practice being more positive, and Meditate, find quiet time to reconnect with the whisper of Spirit or God within and Share your gifts with others.

I know that you are an Audrey Hepburn admirer, too. You share a common background with your early experience as a ballet dancer. Do you see a correlation there? I know ballet involves much disciplinary work. Do you find discipline is one of the most important factors that add to a sense of well-being?

Michiko: I am honored to share a passion for dance, the language of the soul, with Audrey Hepburn. Ballet training embodies the idea that the Arts are seen as disciplines. Cultivating discipline is a catalyst that can awaken self-respect, self-love, which manifests as freedom of expression. Ultimately, well-being is the fruit of contentment from exercising soul mastery and sharing our best with others.

Do you feel beauty starts from the inside out? If so, why and how can someone that has been self-conscious about their looks learn to develop a stronger core to feel better about themselves?

Michiko: Mindful Breathing is the master key to feeling better instantly. It not only inspires you, it empowers you to feel strong in your core and beautiful (be you to the fullest) from the inside out. We start with the commitment to seeing ourselves in a whole new diamond light. When you adjust your attitude, to get grounded, gracious and gorgeous, being self-conscious is replaced with 'I Got This' self-confidence. Empower-up Tip: From Korby Banner, Celebrity Photographer and Makeup Artist. He says to be seen as beautiful our whole life, we need these three vital traits:

- Good posture
- Kind eyes
- Genuine smile: I say, "We got this."

When beauty can sometimes feel shallow or vain if we focus on just our skin, it's important to remember to look deeper when finding a natural glow of your own. That does not involve any trips to the plastic surgeon. There are no needles necessary when making a soul connection. Only the courage to find out why you were placed on this earth and what brings you moments of joy, while waking up and facing a new day.

Next, let's find out:

- Tricks that can vastly improve your sense of well-being.
- Evaluation of your relationships with your friends. Quantity or Quality?
- Do you know how to experience a 'Seinfeld like Moment'?
- Examine with me one Hollywood movie that inspired a decade and a billion dollar industry for the person that wrote the script.
- Improve your perspective by power of positive thinking. What exactly did Norman Peale mean by that?
- Do you own an animal? How does this relate to losing wrinkles?
- Why reading FICTION is good for your soul.
- Also, are you building sandcastles to the sky?
- Find out what the THREE SOMETHINGS are and why they will help empower your life.

Chapter 5

Visualize What You Want To Be

Being a woman can be hard you know. Just like anything in life, it's just not that easy. I remember when I was eighteen years old a homeless woman at a Taco Bell shop in San Francisco told me my life would be cursed because I was pretty. Now many years looking back I see what her deep meaning meant behind her baggy, saggy clothes, weathered skin and her ideas of educating this young girl on the world to come. Guess what?

She was... *wrong!* Instead of letting this person plant a seed of wrong thought into my mind, I chose to redirect my thinking toward happier thoughts. Life is what we decide we want it to be. If you think you are in for a difficult climb and you will always turn up with the rotten apples, you are right. So try your best to project strong, healthy thoughts into your future.

Try to visualize what you want now... NOW. Don't think, some day; don't think you don't deserve it. Make it happen by actively seeking this vision in your mind.

This book has three layers to it. You have the Soul/ Health/Beauty. Which part is the most important? They are all equally important because they all three affect your sense of well-being. However, the soul came in at number one for me. The soul, what's in your heart, what you love, what brings you joy...*not* your wrinkles on your face, not some skin cream, not a walk in the park, but taking time to nourish your soul first.

Why?

Because what we see in our mind becomes our reality. Yes, you've heard about those amazing self-help books that guide you back into your inner self so you can conquer what threatens to stop you from finding your true heart's desire. If your true heart's desire is to look young, feel healthy and not be defined by your age, then you need to start with your mind first.

Your thoughts will reflect what you want and feel each day. So in this chapter I want you to learn how to visualize each day. Imagine that perfect reality you are hoping to create. Maybe it's losing weight. Maybe you are shy and you need to move out of your 'quiet self' and discover more social activity. Whatever your mind is hoping to achieve, you must first start by actively cleaning out the cobwebs of doubt and insecurity. Dust off that crummy little voice that tells you, "Who do you think you are to want to achieve that?" "That's impossible." "You're too late in the game for anything amazing to happen for you now." *Not true!*

Do you know how many famous, successful individuals are what you call 'A late bloomer'? So many! From Martha Stewart to Abraham Lincoln, the list is endless. So never allow yourself to squash your own wants and dreams because you think you are too old to start something new. I worked in an expensive art gallery last year and sold pieces of art by some artists that didn't start their career until their mid-fifties. Now they have art sculptures hanging all over the world in private art collections, galleries and in a museum because they had the tenacity and the belief in their dream that their age had nothing to do with them achieving what they wanted to accomplish.

So take this time to look within your heart and discover that hidden gem that might be missing from your life. When you find your passion, you rediscover your youth. When we are happy, we look more vibrant and younger. Some secrets to the fountain of youth are quite easy to recognize. We just need to remember to constantly go within for the answers for what we need. Go within to find that voice that can guide you forward.

The one thing about my life is it shows lots of creativity. Whenever I become complacent, I challenge myself to go within and find something new to inspire me. Let me share with an example of a Hollywood legend that had his pulse on this topic.

Famous movie director John Huston who is best known for *The Treasure of Sierra Madre*, *The Maltese Falcon*, and *The Night of The Iguana*, starring Richard Burton. In the last film I mention, while John Huston was working on location on this particular production, he had asked his cast out to dinner. Then the question was asked, "What makes the world tick?" Many of the cast members said, "Money." However, when they came to John Huston, he paused ever so briefly and then answered simply... *interest*. His answer rings true so deeply with me because if we are not interested or inspired in our lives – at least for me... I began to fall into that 'on automatic' phase where I am waking up and simply going through my routine each day and not challenging myself. Who wants to live only half a life? If we are given this specific life, shouldn't we relish in the joy and discovery of the new?

So please do yourself a favor and before you decide on that expensive facial treatment because the Real Housewives on Bravo just had it done, go within your own soul first to find out how you can shave off the stress, the added years that you feel are starting to reflect in your age. Are you making time for you to have fun? Or are you just constantly clocking in at work and hating the fact you have to do it all over again?

"Change your thoughts and change your world." You know you've heard that quote; Norman Vincent Peale said that. Something like that anyway. I just know that there is so much more to women that just another facial treatment, skin tuck or eye lift. I know there are many wonderful deep souls out there that could be reading this thinking, she doesn't mean me does she? No. I mean the current trend for women to alter their natural appearance with a foreign substance that doesn't belong there in the first place.

Think deeper. Breathe deeper. Don't limit your mind to just the surface. Try harder and discover what gives you joy and what you could be missing that could change your life today. It's never too late to become the person you've secretly wanted to be in your world.

So here are some quick tips on how to visualize your dream so you can make it happen. Maybe the term goal or wish works better for you. The main thing is to VISUALIZE what you want to happen.

- Take time before you go to bed at night and actively color in that blank canvas every detail of how the look and feel of what you want to become or do will feel like. Imagine that it has already happened. Now say a thank you prayer, too, that you have achieved what you are imagining. Set at least five minutes a night before you go to bed so you can actively sink these thoughts deep into your subconscious.
- Begin actions that will build your dream. Hard work will be part of what you are wanting to become. Nothing great is ever achieved without persistence, desire and activity. Maybe your action is writing a plan that you can also read to yourself on your smart phone, in between quiet moments of your day. Focus your thoughts whenever you can on that wish and see it firmly in your mind.
- Tell someone you trust about what you want to happen and remind them to keep you inspired.
- Is there someone you can look up to that has already done what you want to do? I am sure there is. So take my advice and find out how they did it. Inspire your mind by seeing how they already MADE their dream materialize.
- Don't give up. Don't be persuaded to quit. Remember to keep your mind active with thought, visualization and prayer in order to activate the changes you want to see in your world. Believe in yourself. Coach yourself and speak kind words always to your dream.

In the quest of Middle Age Beauty we must first discover what we love the most and what gives us that eternal glow that only can come from a deep passion from within our soul. You have the power to become that dream. So start now.

After all, it is up to you to forge ahead and become your own best intentions. Make sure you are visualizing the best for yourself always. World famous philosopher James Allen said it best, "Dreamers are the *Saviors* of the world." Not all of my dreams have always come true. But goodness, I've had so much fun trying so many different things on this journey.

Chapter 6

Find Time To Make New Friends

I'm one of those women that just loves her girlfriends! I love having as many as possible from all different age groups. A lover of communication and the soul makes 'girl chat' time fun and worthwhile in my life. You might remember I have it listed as one of my joyful moments on my list of my joyful things to do every day. Do you have lots of friendships? If you do, then this chapter should be one you read through *carefully*. Magazines from *Woman's Day* to many other blogs and online forums that have lists like:

Top Ten reasons friendships are important.

I love titles like this. I know many of the reasons just like you do on why it's important to have girlfriends.

Here are my top three:

- They are fun! It's wonderful to meet up with other women to find out what's going on in their lives.
- We have another voice with an opinion that is a female feeding us insight that can be eye opening and decisive when we cannot be.
- Sharing your life with others makes it so much more exciting.

These are obvious facts that we all know without reading a list online or in a magazine. This chapter is asking you to do one more step, which will be important for the health of your soul and protecting that vulnerable eyebrow section that tends to wrinkle when we worry and fret. What do women worry about besides babies, men and their family?

Friendships! Unfortunately the example of women being

friends on reality shows that filter our nightly living can be ultimately frightening. Is that really the way women are? I'm actually giving those women the benefit of the doubt. If I happen to catch one of those 'housewives' shows, I am hoping that most of this is being instigated by the producers and not truly 'reality!'. Right?

Because if so, just we women as a species may be headed for trouble. It would be wonderful to have a reality show depicting friendships of a deeper kind that base their love, honesty and soulful connection on being supportive and loving versus the cat-fighting antics and competitiveness. Where is that group of women?

I know what you are thinking. We had them in *Sex in the City*. I believe this is why this show had such an international appeal to many. Who wouldn't want three friends that they had brunch with every weekend to recap their woes and tribulations with before facing the next week?

I know I would. In order to love and accept, one must open their heart and share more.

Now, I will be the first to tell you I have had my heart broken by my girlfriends on occasion. Who hasn't? However, when does a friend cross the line when their opinion begins to be critical and judgmental of your soul?

Here are the facts:

Life is short
No one is perfect
Be happy now
Choose your friends wisely

Why is that last statement so important? Well because if your friend is one of those that constantly critically discusses with you your personality flaws or *what you need to work on as an individual*, then you might want to consider looking for a new friend or clique to hang out with... why? Because criticism is different than constructive criticism. Your friends are not your psychiatrists. They do not have a PhD in Psychology (or maybe they do!) and life is tough enough without someone you love jabbing you on a daily basis with ugly words that can feel like a sucker punch in the middle of the day after you click off your cell phone.

Here is a quick quiz for you to determine and measure your friendships:

Do you look forward to talking to your girlfriend or do you have that 'pit' feeling in your stomach like you might be getting chewed out soon?

A. Yes

B. Never

C. Maybe

Would you trust their influence with your child? If you aren't a mother, feel free to insert a nephew or niece to this equation.

A. Yes

B. Never

C. Maybe

Do you start to doubt yourself more after you hang out with them or speak to them on the phone?

A. Yes

B. Never

C. Maybe

Do you feel competitive with them over the phone or in person?

A. Yes

B. Never

C. Maybe

Do you think your friend could handle the truth if you shared with them something they did that bothered you? Can you truly be your 'real self' with them, or are you trying to be accepted based on merits you think they are seeking in you?

A. Yes

B. Never

C. Maybe

Are you constantly worrying about what your friend might think?

A. Yes

B. Never

C. Maybe

This is not a pass or fail test. This is for you to check in with yourself and see how you feel about your friend or friendships. If any of your answers were a definitive negative answer to the question, then you are ready for this next part of the chapter on my advice on how to find friends, what to do with the trouble-makers and why it's more fun to have as many as possible versus just ONE best friend.

If friendships can be challenging, why have more?

This answer is fairly simple. The more friends you have, the more flexibility you will have as a friend and a person. Obviously, you are going to have a few closer friends with deeper meaning, that mirror and affect your soul in such a positive fashion that after you speak to them you feel like you just had a dose of sunshine and a quick shot of espresso.

Best Friends are great. But trust my advice and make more. You might be missing out on a golden friendship of a lifetime if you only stick with the ones you have always known.

My girlfriends are great. Are yours?

Where to search for new girlfriends to add to your Friendship Pot

Don't worry, I'm not going to suggest Bingo on Friday night. But, hey if that's big in your town go for it! This quest is always challenging for us all in life because it requires us to move out of our comfort zone and 'put ourselves out there'. It's not always easy exposing our souls. Well, don't think of it like that.

Friendship is sort of like peeling an onion. One layer at a time to get to the core. So just know that when meeting in new settings it is good to protect your more vulnerable self until you can identify who is trustworthy.

Here are a few examples of where you can mingle to find the next best friendship you never knew existed:

- Join a book club. So you don't like to read. So what? Push yourself to do that when joining a group through a bookstore or check with the library in town, too.
- Try church or an organized group in your community. Talk about one place you can walk into and almost guarantee you won't be nervous – attending a ceremony at any church in your neighborhood. Of course, you go to church for other reasons first. Join a women's Bible study group. (If you aren't religious, you can still join to find some new friends.) You never know, this experience might be the beginning of a beautiful friendship.
- Take a dance class. Dancing already is one of those keys to getting in touch with your soul. Look online or on a cork billboard at your local community gathering area. Dance away, while keeping an eye out for a new friend.
- Julia Child anyone? Yes, obvious to many and maybe it sounds cliché, but joining a cooking class reminds me of that fun movie Nora Ephron wrote *Julie and Julia* based on two books: one involving Julie Powell, and Julia Child's memoirs. This not only sounds like an adventure, but also a sure way to meet other women (or men!) that could become your new friends who will be calling you daily for your cooking secrets. Did you know that if you Google Julia Child's name 55,200,000 sites pop up? Wow that's incredible! Julia rocked the Middle Age Beauty group with her true authentic self!

So remember that having more friends in life gives you more options, more fun time and a chance to learn more from others. Relationships are a key ingredient to watering our soul. Just make sure you are surrounding yourself with the right types of friends. If you need a therapist, pay for one. Don't be bullied and beaten by critiqued conversations from someone that may just really want to sabotage your inner light.

What to do with the Trouble Makers

Okay. So you aren't ready to part with that one friend you may be reevaluating right now in your mind. But could this friend be treading slightly on your inner confidence? So what to do? Are you not ready for the ax to swing and to cut off all ties? How to mend the fence with your friend:

- Set new boundaries.
- Spend less time with them.
- Think positive thoughts about your friendship and evaluate your own actions regarding why the friendship is starting to sour.
- Be nicer. You never know, your friend might be going through a hard time and concealing it from you. So always offer the white rose just in case you haven't been informed of a major upset that could be causing the issues. Let time do its own healing naturally. Don't worry. If you are real friends, a mini-break won't damage the relationship.

Friendships are worth investing in, worth finding and also, guess what? So much fun! *So make time to find time to be a friend and have friends.* After all, you could be that someone special to someone else that truly values the real *you*. So what is the one thing you are going to do again? *Make room for one new friend.*

Chapter 7

Moments Like Seinfeld

When I lived in Los Angeles during the 90s there was a brief period where I performed at The Comedy Store on the Sunset Strip in 'The Belly Room' with an improv comedy troupe. This is different than standing up doing a solo act, which I feel most everyone associates with comedy.

Improv is when you work with a group of people and perform a scene from scratch, building it out of the organic moment of *Now*. One rule that struck me to be an interesting rule of improv is the rule to always say 'yes and' to build what you were going to add to the scene. You were never allowed to say no because there would be nowhere for the scene to build.

If you are always saying yes to life with a smile, what could be better than that? Well, that's how my brief encounter with comedy felt, magical and fun. Oh, trust me, comedy is one of the hardest things I've ever done as far as feeling brave and being brave when it comes to things like stage fright.

George Milner said that: *"laughter breaks us up when we are being too extreme or taking ourselves too seriously."* Life is about not knowing, having to change, taking the moment and making the best of it, without knowing what's going to happen next.

Just like in comedy, when it comes to our soul in order to find a balance of seriousness, discipline and heart, trust me, one of the most important things you can do in life is just this:

Have Some Fun

When we allow ourselves to connect with the silliness that can allow us to 'cut loose' and let go, we are without realizing it relaxing our bodies and connecting to that inner child that just wanted to enjoy summer vacation. Silly moments like these are worth working for each week. Just ignore those beauty ads of how old we are getting, and do take pity on those young actresses who have had countless surgeries during their early twenties.

Really?

Is life coming to this for women? Young women are going under the knife to feel better about themselves, rather than looking within to connect with that scary stuff that actually might make them feel something.

Connecting to your soul through silly moments can come in many different forms. You don't have to join an improv group to experience a 'Seinfeld Moment'. You don't have to make a fool of yourself either in order to obtain moments of bliss.

The trick is to allow yourself first to RELAX. Don't take yourself so seriously. So what. You are over forty. Stop judging yourself and comparing how you look to those reality stars on Bravo. This is about you. This is about having the courage to stop being so uptight when you are in a group of friends in order to feel accepted.

Dare To Be Funny

Make someone laugh by sharing a funny story. Add a quirky dynamic to your circle of friends by spreading joy instead of gossip. Who cares who had what procedure done last week, who weighs more, which house has the most square footage and what accolades your child has achieved in sports. Have some fun and let loose with your friends. Laugh a little.

This is one of my favorite things to do. My girl time. I tend to maybe go overboard on making those around me laugh because I enjoy so much hearing others sharing in the laughter, too. The trick it is to STOP taking yourself too seriously.

Trust me, if you are too pompous to come off your high horse and never allow yourself to look or feel silly moments, you are missing an important connection that could be adding much happiness to your daily life with yourself and your other relationships.

I'm sure you have heard that famous quote, "Dance like no one is watching." I say *dance like everyone is watching and enjoy it.* Enjoy experiencing connecting with your silly side while hanging with your peer group.

I once had a friend tell me regarding another girlfriend, "She is just going to break your heart. I would not get too close to her." "Really?" I responded. "If she does, at least I experience something real instead of holding back and playing it safe." That is what comedy is about. That is what improv is about. And risking being silly in front of those you love, just to kick up the room temperature with some much needed fun, is one payoff you will never regret.

Okay, you say, *"I don't have a clue how to connect with a silly side. That's just not me."* Well, fine. Stop reading this chapter and skip to the cheap beauty products. If you just want to continue on as a person that is so serious you can't even relax enough to make someone else feel good, you don't deserve to connect to that inner child that longed for summer moments away from the discipline of school. If you can let your hair down to relax and find some time to have some fun, well maybe read ahead to the health part so you can figure out how to apply your seriousness to your health since that is such an important part of the equation to the beauty trinity, too.

In all seriousness though, your soul is the number one part of this book. Your soul needs to feel like: *"Hey, this is awesome, life is pretty good. I want to have some more fun today."* Trust me, you will stop concentrating on new wrinkles forming or what face filler to use next because your mind and heart and soul are AWAKE from being jubilantly exuberant from just cutting loose for a few moments.

Am I making my point here? There is a reason why *Seinfeld* will go down in history as one of the most memorable sitcoms in the history of television. Even though it was a 'show about nothing', Elaine, Jerry, Kramer and George were sure having some fun in the meantime.

Here are my suggestions for you to make time for some more smile lines than furrowing the little spot right between your eyebrows. This is building on the meditation, which teaches you how to relax, breathe deeper and to empty your mind.

Now it's time to fill in the dots, say No to Botox and yes to learning some exercises that connect us to that inner child that's dying to laugh a little today. Think less about aging and more about experiencing some fun moments.

How to jump-start your Funny Bone:

- Sing out loud loudly. Maybe in the shower or in your car, but connect those vocal cords to your feelings and watch the stress begin to role off your shoulders.
- Turn up the music in your home. Dance really ridiculously and bad. So badly you can't even believe you are doing such silly things. Trust me, it feels good to express the 'Silly part of your soul'.
- If your day is feeling crummy and you can't seem to muster up any joy, FAKE IT. You can fool yourself into feeling happy. I do this all of the time. I have to admit what happens is I begin to laugh at myself for the extreme measures I am taking to feel blissful!
- Be somewhat self-deprecating. Think of Ellen and her crazy dance. Trust me, there is a reason why Ellen is so successful. Yes, she is funny, but she knows how to dance in front of us all without missing a beat. You can tell she's having fun on her show, which makes her contagious to watch as a viewer. Make up your own silly dance and express yourself!
- Bop your head up and down to the music, while you are driving. I know. Hey, throw in a shoulder move that has

you pulling a vogue moment like Madonna.

- Tap your feet in the office quietly. Hear a song in your mind and dance to the beat of the song in your imagination. Believe in fun times each day.

Just like the lyrics suggest, *Tonight's Gonna Be a Good Night* by the Black Eyed Peas, jump up and bounce some during your hectic schedule. Bounce, groove, stick your tongue out, make a fool of yourself to yourself. Dare to fall out of the serious Poser's Group and relax a bit. Country music star Reba McEntire said these three bones are essential:

To succeed in life you need three things: a wishbone, a backbone and a funny bone.

I love laughing. I love feeling silly. I love being relaxed. I love having my own Seinfeld like moments because life is too short to miss out on a smile I might have missed if I didn't take the leap of faith and risk looking ridiculous. After all, your soul deserves a good laugh on who? *You!*

Chapter 8

Are You In Touch with Your Leadership Skills?

You may not know this either because I didn't before I interviewed Dr. Anthony F. Smith. Did you know women are better leaders than men? Yes, we've all heard that and secretly wondered, *"If that's so, why are there more men as CEOs than women in business?"* How can this fact be possible and is it a fact or an opinion? I must say I wondered this before I sat down with Dr. Anthony F. Smith, the author of *Taboos of Leadership*, and the co-founder and Managing Editor of Leadership Research Institute. LRI specializes in leadership development and assessment for companies around the world. Working with large companies like the Walt Disney Company, ESPN and Coca-Cola – just to name a few – Dr. Anthony F. Smith has devoted his life to discovering what makes better leaders. In his book, he uncovers in secret number four, "Women Make Better Leaders (When That's What They Really Want to Do)". How wonderful to hear such a positive affirmation for women at any age. I had to get to the bottom of this and find out just how women excel in the field of leadership.

Here is my candid one on one interview with Dr. Anthony F. Smith:

In your book *Taboos of Leadership*, Secret 4 states that women make better leaders than men in business? Can you expand upon the philosophy of that a little here?

Dr. Anthony F. Smith: This isn't my personal opinion. This is based on scientific evidence and the qualities of what makes a great leader. There are leaders and there are followers in all areas of life. In the US today the greater the diversity spectrum from gender to ethnicity, the greater the challenges become for the leader to influence. You have to be a cognitive thinker and more diverse as a leader. Now women are more adaptable because they are holistic thinkers... which literally means 'whole brain thinking'. Now how does science prove this? What is the one difference between men and women? The corpus callosum which binds our left and right brain hemispheres together is *larger* for women. Now why are there not more leaders in business as there are men? Women are more relationship driven, while men are more success driven. When women are getting close to becoming the top executives of companies, a majority of women don't make the next leap in business because what is a priority to them is not climbing the corporate ladder.

You referenced Mother Teresa as an example of a powerful world leader before our interview started. Why do you think Mother Teresa was able to transcend the barriers of religion? Do you think that her gender factored into this equation?

Dr. Anthony F. Smith: Women are more compassionate and empathic. They are more demonstrative with their emotion. While men are taught not to show their feelings. Also Mother Teresa had a mission that drove her to help the poor and needy all over the world. Nothing would separate her from this mission. So yes I do believe that her gender played a significant role in why she was such a powerful world leader.

You have worked with companies like ESPN, Disney and Coco-Cola and many others over a span of twenty years. Your background and education is impressive. How did you discover that women make better leaders than men? Was it by working with so many different executives and companies over the last 20 years?

Dr. Anthony F. Smith: Well, both. The scientific evidence was there to back up this evidence and part of my job as a consultant is to help leaders adapt and change during trying and economic times. Women are more open and better listeners than men. They also tend to leverage the capabilities of others better because they are more of a collaborator and less ego driven... To be a leader, you don't have to be submerged in the corporate world. There are many forms of leadership. From running a household, to a position at a church or like Dr. Martin Luther King, Jr., who we know was one the most influential leaders of our time. There are many great examples for women leaders like Oprah Winfrey to Indra Nooyi the CEO of PepsiCo. Many of them you may not know their names. But take a look at Forbes Fortune 500 to find out who some of these amazing women are that are the top CEOs of the world.

How important is it for someone to trust their inner voice from their soul when it comes to their work environment? Do you feel there is a link between the two?

Dr. Anthony F. Smith: In my books I talk a lot about listening to your inner voice when it comes to business. You often hear stories about regrets in business, when someone says, "I wish I would have done this instead of that," when they knew from the beginning that was the right choice. Great leaders trust their intuition and follow that inner voice. Now when you look at what intuition is, some may think it's spiritual but most could say from a logical standpoint that intuition – or that inner voice – is derived from pattern recognition over a period of time. Here's why. Pattern recognition demands exquisite observational skills. Now guess who is better at that when it comes to men and women? Yes, that's right, a woman.

What advice could you give women who are over forty and looking to begin again with a new career choice, knowing they have excellent leadership skills?

Dr. Anthony F. Smith: Don't think that you have to become more masculine and male to exercise your leadership abilities. Why women fail sometimes is they try to mimic their male counterparts. Now that does not mean they shouldn't try and fit into a masculine surrounding. But don't give up your own natural leadership abilities to become someone else, because women are amazing collaborators and lastly make sensational leaders.

Wow, I must say after my interview with Dr. Anthony F. Smith I walked a little taller out to my car that day. I found myself asking how I could become a better leader in my own circumstances, which boils down to wife, mother, writer and entrepreneur. I felt inspired to know these new brimming facts that females just rock at leadership. So ask yourself and apply these questions to your life. If you have excellent leadership skills, how can you apply this knowledge to your world? How can you empower yourself to become the natural born leader you already are?

In a world that can demean us still because we are women, it's good to hear information like this. It's important to know that being a female doesn't mean we are just the Trophy Wife, The Mommy that makes the meals and shuttles the kids around to their events. You are leading your family. You are making an important mark with your own personal relationships. So take great pride in the different areas of where you can identify yourself as the 'Leader of the Pack'.

Also, is there something you've always wanted to do but you may think you are too old now? You may be thinking, "It's too late in the game of life for me to try something new."

Throw those negative thoughts out the window!

Some of the most successful examples of leaders in history and today are what some might call 'late bloomers'. Julia Child, Grandma Moses, Colonel Sanders, Andrea Bocelli and Harrison Ford are some famous late bloomers that hit their stride later in life. So don't make excuses. Find a focus, a dream or a passion that sets your soul on fire to redefine who you are again.

I personally love to change up my scenery often when it comes to my work environment. From working as an actress, a model, to selling expensive masterpieces in an art gallery, I have had so much fun challenging myself to explore and do many different things. You don't have to run out and quit your day job either. I have one successful girlfriend living in Los Angeles right now that was just nominated for an Emmy as a successful set designer. However, her passion is also in accessories, jewelry and sharing her love for this with her friends. So now she has become a representative for a classy jewelry line and hosts many fabulous parties with her friends, while making extra money. Some might think, why would she do that when she was just nominated for an Emmy in set design? Because that's what's driving her heart and passion in her soul.

You don't have to become the CEO of a corporate business to feel successful or empowered from your soul. You just need to connect within and find what gives you that extra sparkle to add zest to your schedule. Remember, *be creative.*

Take this time right now to jot down a few ideas of what you've always wanted to try, but haven't.

This is an example of what the list might look like:

- Painting classes.
- Dance class.
- Creative writing class.
- Fitness training work.
- Start a side business with a partner.
- Go back to school to learn some new business courses that could help you become more savvy in the workforce.
- Take an online college course you've always wanted to take but thought you couldn't because of your age.

So don't make any excuses for yourself. You have the natural capacity to achieve greatness with certain scientific positives that you were given for just being a woman. Don't sell yourself short ever because of your sex. Don't foresee any obstacles in your way. Make a plan. Write it down and apply that natural leadership skill that is just brimming to be shared with the world. Remember to say only kind words with positive affirmations in your mind. Donald Trump just said recently, *"Remember, if you don't promote yourself, then no one else will! Likewise, believe in yourself – or no one else will either."*

Chapter 9

Be Optimistic with Your Thoughts

During my mid-twenties you could say I had an early midlife crisis. When upon reaching the age of 25, my life felt uncertain and somewhat empty. Being from a small town in Missouri, most of my friends had already gotten married and had children.

When I turned 25 I awoke to find myself living alone in an A-frame cabin in Studio City where the walls were so thin, my dad joked I was living in a 'Lean-to' out in Los Angeles. Well, looking back, he was pretty much right on the money. Well, it was a beautiful little cottage surrounded by a bricked-in courtyard with lots of charm. I think that's how a realtor would say it.

Anyway, it's not exactly the picture I had in mind when I was 25. I was just shocked at where I had landed. What to do when life feels wrong? Shift your thinking and figure out why. So if you are living right now in your middle-aged lifetime wishing you were still twenty and hating each birthday with your passing age, you are just setting yourself up for failure.

Rule number one. Remember? "Don't lie about your age." Why? Because aging is a gift. Many are not fortunate to live a long life. If you are, don't hate yourself because of a birthday. Don't define who you are because of a number. Don't buy into the shallowness and falsified lives of those reality show ladies that are showcasing their life to make money. (I am sure some of them are lovely women, too.) Remember, what you are watching is after all entertainment and *not* their real life.

What is their real life like? Who Cares? Let's get your life on track and figure out why so many women have a problem with turning forty and are pumping their faces full of fillers...

Okay. So how did I make it past my early midlife crisis?

I prayed.

That's right. I asked for guidance. I sought counsel and I found out that my *thoughts* were incredibly wrong and I began to refocus my mind. I look back and see myself in that tiny cabin living out in Hollywood all by myself and I have to smile at my bravery.

Luckily for me, I had a wonderful grandmother that sent these little pamphlets in the mail to help me learn how to shift my thinking. My mentor and friend also had a great quote she shared with me:

The key to relaxation is simple: we must monitor doubt and constantly refocus to stay positive.
~ Michiko Rolek

Just because my friends were all married with children did not make me a failure. So remember to stop comparing yourself to an 'idea' of what you think your life should look like.

Here are three simple rules to follow when activating positive thinking:
Rule number one:
Stop comparing your life to your friends.
Rule number two:
Remember to redirect your thinking to positive energy when self-doubt begins to hover in your mind.
Rule number three:
Wake up with the attitude that life is going your way today.

I guess in some ways I was lucky to feel the number crunch early on. I learned at a decent age that my AGE was just going to keep adding up and there was nothing that I could do about it. When you struggle against reality you cause inner turmoil to your soul.

I have a friend that just told me this: "I'm not afraid of much in my life except my birthdays." This I think is a common theme among women. Count me in as one of them. I felt that way, too, until I did some redirecting of my thoughts and found out why wishing for what can never happen will only bring you inner turmoil. Never struggle against reality. To wish for what cannot be can only bring you strife in any set of circumstances.

So when I was 25 I did some investigating. I figured out and calculated why I was staring up at this wooden A-frame ceiling.

I figured out how I had arrived there. I remembered being a model at a young age, which led me to live in subsequent cities in the United States and finally landed me in Hollywood, since my looks were more commercial. I listened to my agents tell me to try acting because there was money in commercials. So I did that, too. I had just broken up with a boyfriend because I realized that maybe our personalities didn't really bring out the best in each other. So there I was 25 and feeling like life was over for me. Unmarried and unloved… what could be worse at 25?

I am semi-kidding here. Although that was exactly how I felt then. Remember life is not perfect. Those with the marriage or the bigger house may be wishing to be where you are if you are footloose, single and free. So stop comparing yourself to your friends. Do inventory on *why* you feel the way you do and do something about changing your thinking.

Redirect your steps. Once I realized that getting married and having children were at the forefront of my wish list, I made a promise to myself to go on that path and make that happen. I began to study these little pamphlets that my Grandmother Lula would send me, about "The Power of Positive Thinking."

Norman Vincent Peale (yes, I have mentioned him before and will probably mention him a few times in this book) was a famous pastor who also is known for writing one of the first self-help books. His method to his principles was quite simple really. Change your thoughts, and imagine what you want to be, and then fuel that with taking action. Be Big, Think Big and Act Big. Discover Enthusiasm. Feel Joy. Live the life you were meant to live and also discover what makes you happy.

He had a simple rule in one of his books, "Act as if and you will Be." Now what exactly does that mean? Let me break it down into simple terms for you: FAKE IT. Hey, I don't wake up every day naturally happy. Most of us don't. However, I also don't just sit around and wait for the mood to strike me either. I consciously work my way by 'acting as if' I am happy. Eventually, after a strenuous effort, I am feeling more optimistic, pleasant and finding that smile. Try it.

This man revolutionized my life into simple principles that work because he believed that *God had indeed wanted us to find some joy now, and not just sit around and wait for Heaven.* (If you are agnostic, I am sure you get the drift here.)

Norman Vincent Peale capitalized heavily on the principle that we as individuals have the power to harness our mental power and change our lives. Life was not just a feeling. Life could be a directed path with clear, concise thoughts that can activate our joy and daily livelihood. To just think positive was only the beginning. The philosophy he taught behind his many successful self-help books were filled with exercises and actions we must take in order to make the positive thinking take effect on our lives.

So here I am now at the age of 41. I now know what it means to understand the power of my own thoughts, the power of positivity and how that connects to the happiness in my soul. No longer do I struggle as much with my age, even though I am continuously reminded by ads, television, and ridiculous shows that tell me I need to buy an eyelash enhancer to make my lashes grow longer.

As I revealed in my letter to you in the beginning of this book, I am actively making a choice to embrace this period with enthusiasm. So start celebrating your birthdays with verve and vitality. Believe in the next chapter of your journey with just as much enthusiasm as you did when you were younger. You can still be young at heart. You don't have to be 25 to feel like that age. It's all in your power of cognitive thinking and what you tell yourself.

So what is the message here? Be happy about who and where you are in your life.

You are not over the hill. You can still be young at heart. Start believing in your power of your thoughts and shift your mental power to start working for you today. You are not a desperate housewife. You are young and beautiful in the prime of your journey. So grab on, be bold and shift your thinking to feel more peace of mind in your soul. And if you aren't excited about your current surroundings, you have the power to become the person you still want to be. Maya Angelou, poet and educator said, *"It is this belief in a power larger than myself and other than myself, which allows me to venture into the unknown and even the unknowable."*

Let's go over the key simple ways to activate positive thinking:

- Embrace the 'Act as if' principle and apply that to your life.
- Don't struggle against reality. Embrace the power of your mind and cultivate positive affirmations that can enrich your thinking.
- Memorize key phrases that inspire you. Norman Vincent Peale suggested memorizing key Bible verses to empower your day.

Remember that if you are lucky enough to turn one year older, that you have been blessed with your current age. Life can be incredibly short. So learn to accept aging while staying young at heart. After all, do *think positive* and believe in your future.

Chapter 10

Soul Mate? Yes or No?

In our quest for happiness, one of the most important choices we make will be the person we choose to spend our lives with at the end of the day. Maybe you are not a big believer in marriage and you just want to stay in a relationship without the ring. Maybe you are married right now and wondering if you married the right person? Maybe you are single or newly divorced and thrust back into the single world. Either way, this is the big question that at some point we will all have to face: your life partner.

My life has been a quest for that off and on. I must admit at an early age I believed in 'happily ever after'. It's not that I don't believe in that or believe in my current relationship, but for now I try most desperately to be thankful for the 'now'. I love my husband. He is amazing. He is like one of those types of men you look for your whole life and discover later on because you are able to recognize him. Do you know what I mean by that? I married my husband at the age of 38. I had to live a few lifetime experiences to actually understand and appreciate all of Robin's wonderful attributes besides the fact he is quite handsome. I don't want to bore you with an 'in love story', that might bore you to tears; but what I do want to do is to help you recognize what you do deserve in a relationship. I'm not one of those women that are going to tell you to marry the rich guy. I am the type of woman to tell you stay single or become single if you are with someone that doesn't treat you with kind words, encouragement or take time to encourage you to believe in your dreams.

So many times women buy into that time-ticking clock that forces them maybe to marry or seek a relationship so they do not fall into the category of becoming 'single' forever. Inevitably, after the cake has been sliced into many pieces and the dress stored in a box in the attic, real life does set in. So make sure that you can live amicably with the person you choose. Make sure that this person is someone that believes in you. Many times attraction and love are not enough. I am asked often if am 'in love' with my husband.

If you happen to be a close girlfriend of mine you would know that answer is yes. I married a man that brings out the best in me. He sees my dreams as tangible, worthwhile projects. He never tells me I need to lose weight or hey baby, "Can you just stop talking to me for awhile and call one of your girlfriends?" Why? Because he is my best friend. I love to hang out with him. I just like being in his presence. I would compare the way I feel to the way Katherine Hepburn felt about Spencer Tracy. She was a trailblazer for independent women during an era where wearing trousers or slacks was considered a controversy. Her independent spirit seemed to be just out of reach for even the infamous Howard Hughes to capture as his own. She was her own woman... until she met Spencer Tracy. After that, she spent her life with his wants and needs more important than her own.

That's happened to me with Robin, my husband. If someone would have told me twenty years ago that love would come in the form of a produce/gift shop in Rancho Santa Fe, I would've been too naïve to believe them. I also had more illusions attached to what I thought would make me happy versus knowing when you follow your soul's heartbeat everything will fall into place naturally. I would've never believed that dipping chocolate berries could be so satisfying or talking to people about avocados could feel so wonderful. But when you are in love these things become a 'side item' of the person you are sharing their world with and you are just grateful to see their face every night before you go to bed.

I hope that we stay married and the future welcomes us with love. We will strive to grow stronger as a couple, more in love each year. But for now, I will say thank you for my blessings and continue to be grateful for the *now*.

Sometimes we want to pinpoint a relationship as a 'forever thing', like you will be with this one person for many years. The facts are we cannot predict life. All you can do is try to grab on now to what's in front of you. So take my advice. Open your eyes to the person that treats you with respect and make sure you have feelings for them, too. Don't fall for the 'bad boyfriend type' that you have an attraction for... meanwhile they treat you like an afterthought. If the person you are spending your daily routine with is saying ruthless, mean words that break your soul down into a lifeless zombie, then it's time to say goodbye! Find the courage to be alone and live for something wonderful that could be existing in the near future.

If you happen to be married to this person, seek counsel first. Is there something to save? Were you ever in love? Do try to see if you can find out where the negativity is coming from within them with a therapist's help.

If this person continues to beseech your soul, do yourself a favor – find some courage and walk away. It's always best to be alone than in a detrimental relationship that can do some harmful effects to the soul.

So the question is do soul mates exist? My answer to you is…
YES!

I just happen to believe though there could be a few out there existing and your happiness is not just attached to one individual. Moreover, what this book seeks first is to help you find your own amazing self-worth in the prime of your life. Your attachment to someone needing to love you back should never define who you are or what your world looks like.

Before I married for the second time, I was single for eight years. I was a divorced mother during my mid-thirties. I stopped looking and had some 'me time'.

I was engrossed in my own self-discovery, and having some much needed fun with my girlfriends when I wasn't busy raising my son. I sometimes think I found my husband because I simply stopped looking for him. You know that old saying about the pot boiling on the stove. The same is true with relationships.

Here are some important factors you should consider before entering into a permanent relationship with a new partner:

- Are you having fun in the relationship?
- Do they make you believe in the best part of you, your dreams, or your future dreams to come?
- Do your lifestyles mesh? Do you like spending time with this person... as much as you can?
- Do they say kind words to you?
- Do you feel motivated to inspire them to be the best person they can be?
- Do you enjoy being together without other friends around?
- Do you find yourself wanting to make their world a nice place without expecting anything in return?

If you can answer yes to most of these questions, you have found a marvelous match. Take my advice and don't let someone else grab them just because you might not be ready to settle down or are more career oriented at the moment. A perfect fit is impossible to find, but if you do happen to find someone that is also willing to put up with your idiosyncrasies and still build castles to the sky, at least by all means be cognizant enough to not let them slip through your fingers.

Life is a short journey that we are able to create on our own or with the right partner. Just make sure that the person you spend time with isn't some belligerent person that spouts off mean words. Because you would definitely be better on your own, and find the courage to find a person that cares more deeply for your soul. Here is quote for you to ponder. After all, love yourself first, so you can recognize when love knocks knowingly at your door.

To love someone is to understand each other, to laugh together, to smile with your heart and to trust one another. One important thing is to let each other go if you can't do this together.
~ Anonymous

Chapter 11

Create a 'Rocky Like Moment' Three Times a Week

One of the facts in life that we all face is with routine and schedules we can experience dull and boring times. Sometimes it might even feel like the same thing over and over again. If you can relate to this statement or feel you have been there then this chapter is for you. This chapter is for all of us to remember the greatness that exists inside of our souls if we just give ourselves small achievements to work for each week.

Do think prizefighter here. Do think Rocky Balboa from the movie that became famous in 1976. Think about that character Sylvester Stallone created. The one that had the odds stacked against him, including his status in society, his pocketbook, and including his age. A window of opportunity was presented to this fictional character and he managed to muster up the willpower to show up for himself when the bell rang in the ring. We watched Rocky climb the stairs in Philadelphia as the sunrise sparkled off on the horizon.

This movie lead to many more movies. Rocky became a movie legend. An icon, a music theme set with trumpets sounding in perfect unison behind one man that was down and out, but had a dream. Overall from 1976 to current day, the *Rocky* movies created by Sylvester Stallone have grossed over one billion dollars.

Of course this is fiction you say. There are others that are worth mentioning that would make more sense to share than a character that was never even real. This is to showcase an example and a mental picture that you can grasp in your mind. You can visualize the character in his gray sweats climbing the staircase early in the morning. You can hear the music soaring, during the vignettes of training, of the trumpets playing in unison behind the fighter with a dream. The odds were against Rocky. But that didn't stop him from giving his best performance.

Are you giving your best performance in your life? Do you have moments that feel like little victories of success, which make you feel glad you applied your will, strength and gumption toward a goal or an achievement?

If you don't, there is no time like the present to become energized and inspired. Just like this book introduces the beauty trinity, I am encouraging you to design and create three 'Rocky like Moments' a week.

That means achieving three goals during your seven-day calendar. Think of small achievements that you can weave into your schedule that will give you the sensation like the trumpets are sounding, like when Rocky climbed those steps in Philadelphia. Did you know there is a statue there now depicting the prizefighter Rocky holding his hands held high as a symbol of experiencing a moment of self-victory? This can be your little victory, too. You can achieve moments that set your week on fire and motivate you to feel more in sync, more alive in each day by creating your own 'Rocky like Moments'.

Now if you don't want to become a prizefighter, don't worry, that is not what I am suggesting. I am suggesting that you personally discover what sends goose bumps up your spine. Don't you want to feel as glorious as Rocky Balboa did in the movie when he flung his arms up toward the sky?

Do you ever have moments like this? I can tell you that I had to make my own moments up during my week to feel this kind of victory moment, too. I went as far as even downloading the theme song to *Rocky* so I could hear the trumpets sound when I am running my few miles during my neighborhood run.

The trick in life at any age is to stay inspired. We need to create our own inspiring moments to live for each day. Think what we might have missed without scheduling in our proud moments! So remember, your weekly schedule can remain busy and hectic without any time for a few moments of glory. So do what?

Schedule Three Rocky Like Moments A Week!

According to the Macmillan Dictionary the definition 'glory' means: *admiration and praise that you receive because you have done something impressive.* This visual of Rocky Balboa climbing the stairs while he fights for something greater in his life can be used to motivate your own mind. Imagine something you wish to attain, think or do.

Here are a few examples of what some of my weekly 'Rocky Like Moments' look like during my schedule:

- Make a six am spin class at the gym.
- Devote time to painting. (I wish I could do more of this!)
- Run an extra mile during my workout.
- Finish a writing project that I dreaded doing.
- Wake up earlier before my day starts so I can make time to meditate.
- Follow a healthy diet each week when I would rather eat bonbons.
- Read and make time for a good book.

As you can see, these are not all related to working out. Yet they are all based on small actions that I can work for each week. These small actions will help me attain a moment of pride so I can lift my hands above my head in shining achievement.

Midlife time should be more of a sacred and special time for women. Our well-being and attitude are reflected on our expression that we wear every day. Are you reflecting youth and vitality by accomplishing a little 'Rocky Moment' each week? Or are you counting the years and the days and dreading each birthday with each passing year? Don't buy into the fluff and that poor attitude of becoming unwanted because of a number on the calendar.

Join a yoga class. Learn to meditate. Learn to create special moments you can achieve by scheduling them in on your calendar. Force yourself to become more creative with your mind, soul, and body.

Make the 'Rocky like Moment' part of your week created by you. What will yours be? Can you schedule time for yourself to feel your own moments of glory? I hope you do. Because you deserve it.

I may never add up to one billion dollars in achievements during my lifetime. I may never climb those real steps that immortalized a fictional character forever as a statue in Pennsylvania. But I can tell you I will fight each week for my own temporary moments of glory. I will strive to create three things, three actions, three small triumphs that could even just be keeping my kitchen extra clean that week.

Spend some time brainstorming on what your achievements could feel and look like during your week. Now write them down. Choose just three each week. Are you ready to climb the steps of victory? Are you ready to schedule time for yourself to feel your own moments of glory?

Chapter 12

The Three Somethings

Have you ever had one of those days where you just wonder to your self, "What's the point?" When we become uninspired, insecure and lose our enthusiasm, it's easy to fall into a gray space when our life loses its meaning. We can easily fall into a trap filled with self-pity and that position of the 'poor me' syndrome. You know when you want others to feel sorry for you because of circumstances out of your control, for the lot you have been cast, for the dent in your car, for the lack of money in your bank account or for the envy or the success of the neighbors across the street that just won $5000.00 a week for life from the Publishers Clearing House sweepstakes.

Why not me? Why do bad things happen to me?

Trust me, I've had these moments, too. I remember one particular period during my early thirties when I went onto a reality show and had just a horrific experience. In my defense, reality shows were still relatively new on the air. I had been an actress in the past and must admit was attracted to three important letters: NBC. Well, without going into the entire backstory, I will tell you basically the goal of the show was to humiliate each contestant, while hooking them up to a lie detector test. I did have fun during parts of the show, but afterwards when I was thrust out the front door back into the real world, I remember experiencing an insurmountable amount of pity for myself. Recently divorced, a single mother with a three year old and my career on the fritz because I was now in my thirties, I felt rather robbed of something valuable. I wanted some sort of vindication, you know. Like when would I get ahead? When would it be my turn? I meandered in this space probably for a good three weeks until I finally I reached onto my shelf of books and began some positive self-help books. I know. You've got the vision of the middle-aged divorcée in her house sweats, sitting cozy by the fire reading a book on how to get her life back on track. Yes. That. Was. Me.

But guess what, some clichés are built on truths. I found much inner solace during this self-reflective time by looking within instead of blaming others for my own mistakes.

I realized and accepted after that experience that sometimes it's important to know 'when to say when'. I had to admit to myself unless I wanted to commit to a life of auditioning and living in Los Angeles, I was now a divorced, single mom raising her son in San Diego. It was time to dig deep within and remember what I loved in my soul, what inspired me and what could I do that would make me feel proud of myself again?

While the reality world has turned some individuals into household names, my experience left me crying on my sofa alone in the dark looking at numerous letters I had handwritten to the producer. I felt so angry I had allowed myself to be on the show – the casting director knew me and had asked me to join the cast. So I did not go seeking this for myself. I felt like I had been… *had.*

I felt so raw by their blatant attempts to try to humiliate me. I was even given a beautiful little diamond necklace in the shape of an M for my name Machel. (All of the girls received one, not just me.) I packed up my necklace and sent it off to the one crewmember that just happened to be the only genuine, sincere person that I met, while I was filming. He had been so kind to try and divert my attention as I stood outside the lie detector room by asking what it was like growing up on a farm in Missouri. I remember thinking that the act in itself stood out as the only real moment I had experienced on that reality show. I am so glad to have given him that little necklace to show him my thank you for just being real to me. Alas, when the show aired my girlfriends thought I was crazy because I had given up my diamond necklace and all of the other contestants still had theirs. Well, they hadn't gone through a ring of fire and back to tell about it either. Of course, that is somewhat of an exaggeration, but at that time that's how I felt. So what were my motivating factors that helped me turn the corner on this low moment?

What are the Three Somethings?

Something To Believe In
Something To Be Proud Of
Something To Inspire You

I learned this specific philosophy from my mom. My mom is a woman that I am so proud of to have as my mother. I don't want to go off track here and start telling you every story of why my mom is so amazing so let me just stick to these facts by applying what she taught me by living her own example.

Something To Believe In

What do you believe in, do you know? Could you define it if you had to in one paragraph? Are you spiritual, do you have faith, do you believe in the goodness of others, do you believe in a specific cause? What do you believe in? If you don't believe in anything that motivates your mind to stay active or in tune with what you feel is important in your soul, you might as well start writing your epitaph for your headstone. At this period for me, when I had to start over and rediscover a direction, I realized I believed in many things. I believed in the goodness this life has to offer, I believed in the kindness of humanity, the light this world can offer and that one experience was really just a small blurb on my journey. I found my faith in God and in my own self again and stopped feeling sorry for myself.

So what if that one little show didn't go well for me; I was a mother, a daughter, a friend, and I was a woman that did not let one negative experience and other failures allow me to fall off the path of staying upbeat and positive. I had many things to believe in; most of all, I discovered I believed in myself. My advice to you is to take some time and write down what you believe in and how that affects your everyday moments. If my entire experience was to meet one genuine person to reveal they had a heart and cared for me during an embarrassing setup on that show, I am so lucky to have met that person! I am so lucky to have experienced an act of kindness from a fellow human being. So don't let life throw you off track. Don't be dismayed by others' success. Go within. Reestablish your steps and find out what you believe in so you can rise above your insecurities.

Something To Be Proud Of

If you don't have something that makes your soul proud from the inside out, then I would suggest you do some intense 'alone time'. Sit with yourself and discover what makes you feel proud and accomplished from within. This is what I do when I need to find that solid footing. I took a look back over my life and remembered that I loved being a writer. I had written a few things, including a three-act play that I had written which had received favorable reviews for the writing. After making this major connection again, I then went about trying to find a business in which I could apply myself and use my writing talents. I soon found myself working in the newspaper business in Southern California writing press releases for my clients. Next followed a social column of my very own that gave me so much joy to write, each and every deadline. I found myself working hard to build my freelance writing career by submitting my stories and writing for different magazines in Southern California.

Do you have something in your life that you have achieved that makes you feel proud and accomplished? Maybe you've always wanted to paint. Maybe you've always wanted to learn Spanish or take a cooking class. You don't have to have a low point to add excitement to your life. My example of my down point with the reality show is to tell you that I too have had some ups and downs. Life is ultimately a challenge. So with each passing year we have to check in with ourselves to make sure we are living and producing the life we want to live. Find your pride and live the dream. If you've always wanted to sign up for a half marathon, do it!

Something To Inspire You

Let's be honest. Everyday life can be monotonous and boring. What can we do to keep life exciting? Find something that inspires you! Do you know what that is or what that looks like to you? For me, I have many things that inspire me. I do. However, one of my greatest pleasures and secret indulgences is reading luxuriously on my bed with a stack of books next to my bed. What truly is an example of something that inspires me? Reading fiction by my favorite authors. This one little extra hobby of mine has been one of my most dependable sources of inspiration throughout my life. I can't tell you how many moments that I've discovered a new book that introduced a new world to me. One fine example is *Lying Awake* by Mark Salzman. I discovered a nun that had visions of the Lord. Later on in the story you find out the nun has a brain tumor, which could be causing her divine visions. The character must face losing what allows her to experience her closest moments to God by having the brain tumor removed. Does she risk losing her gift that gives her peace, which will eventually kill her? Or does this nun choose to have the operation and struggle with what it feels like to be only normal? As a reader you experience her own struggle with faith and what could life be without that gift.

This is a book that inspired my soul deeply. It moved me to tears. I learned from this writer about an aspect of faith, love and devotion. Do we continue to love in a cruel world that can strip us of our gifts? And how do we continue to have faith when we lose what we love most. *Lying Awake* by Mark Salzman beckoned me to ask myself these same questions.

Reading books inspires me to see new adventures in my life and even to redefine who I am. Reading some of Sophie Kinsella's books inspired me to brighten my wardrobe with some fun designer must-haves. Luanne Rice's novels have always shown me to go deeper with my love. Her books ask you to examine what love is about and at what cost are you willing to risk it all for those that matter most? Kate Kerrigan a historical Irish fiction writer takes me back in time to discover what it would be like to be an Irish woman coming to America for the first time in *Ellis Island*. By examining fiction, I can find inspiration, escape, meaning and excitement.

Being inspired today is almost a cliché saying. It's not the trendiest thing. While the world is glued to our smart phones and tablets – there are many new little gadgets to keep our brains occupied – we must actively seek moments of inspiration to add more value to our precious time on this earth. Seek inspiration every day. Make time to be inspired!

Do little things that inspire you each day, even if it's as simple as reading a book. Without inspiration in our lives, we can lose that zestful purpose and meaning. Middle Age Beauty is first getting in touch with who you are on the inside. If you don't know yourself or like yourself very much, please start being kinder to you. Don't be a harsh critic. Don't say negative words to yourself. Be your own best friend. Learn to connect with what brings you joy, pride, inspiration and what you believe in. Take time for you. If women and men took more time caring for their souls first, little things like wrinkle worries almost sound like dribble. After all, don't let the surprises slow you down too much. I managed to walk away from my acting and modeling career by finding a new world to sink my dreams into. I would have never dreamed that this one could be so much better. Sometimes those lulls and lows are when we find our real inspiration…

Chapter 13

Rescue a Pet

I grew up on a farm in Southern Missouri. My upbringing in 4-H showing cattle for blue ribbons at the county fair instilled in me at an early age the importance of animals in my life. Some little girls played with dolls. I played with our many farm cats that kept my heart entertained, loved and fulfilled. When I moved to Los Angeles permanently at the age of nineteen years old, one of the first things I did was visit the Santa Monica Animal Shelter to adopt a kitten for my new journey in California. I then adopted another cat later on, too.

You couldn't really call me the crazy cat lady yet because I am a little young for that and I don't have that many, but only two. I will tell you that during some of my darkest hours alone during my twenties when I felt isolated and cut off from my family these two kitties gave me something to care for and to love, which in turn made my foundation as a person just a bit more solid when I lived alone in Los Angeles.

Now here I am twenty-odd years later still with cats and feeling so fortunate to know each one along the way. You might be wondering what in the world adopting a pet could have to do with your beauty, health and soul, so let me get down to some scientific research besides my personal cat stories that might and should persuade you to rescue a pet that needs saving today.

Did you know according to a study done by the Minnesota Stroke Institute cats help fight heart disease, which is the leading cause of death among men and women? Yes, that's right, owning a cat can save your life. The study followed 4,000 cat owners over a period of ten years, monitoring their life and their health versus non-animal owners. Thirty percent of those studied were less likely to die from a heart attack. So stating that owning a cat can save your life is something that should definitely figure into your equation of adopting a pet.

Dogs are just as amazing. I once listened to the personal story of the president of Helen Woodward Animal Center in Southern California relive how he was saved by a dog in New York City on the East Coast. A couple of thugs had knifed a dog and left it to bleed to death in the middle of the street. The two thugs then stood on the side of the road taking bets on how long it would live. Mike Arms came upon the situation and asked the two men why they were not helping the poor bleeding animal. When he found out what had happened he stepped in and scooped the dog up from the street to take him immediately to an animal hospital. But then the worst thing happened. Mike Arms was then attacked by these two men and was left to bleed to death in the street right next to the dog. As he recounted the story to a group of us in Rancho Santa Fe, I silently cried tears listening to what happened next. On the brink of dying, Mike Arms said he regained consciousness by the licking of the dog that was right next to him. He said that dog used his last bit of life to help save him and from that moment on he dedicated his life to helping save animals all over the world. From service dogs that can detect seizures and working dogs that protect soldiers, dogs are indeed man's best friend.

In 2008, CBS reported a story of a six year old boy that couldn't speak. There were no medical reasons for his condition either. However, that all changed when a therapy dog named 'Boo' visited his classroom at school. The first word he spoke was – Boo! The mother soon found out that Boo was the name of a therapy dog that had just been to school. The story ruminates that most adults wouldn't think as much about the tricks done by a therapy dog. However, to the six year old boy, it was like seeing magic that helped him connect to his soul and finally speak for the first time in his life.

This is just one story of many. Animals have the ability to

reach our souls sometimes even when we cannot. They take our minds off of our own wants and needs and bring us into 'the now', which help us live a more mindful, meaningful life.

My recommendations to find a pet:

Check with the local shelter near where you live.

If you are interested in a particular breed, first look for a rescue organization of the breed you are interested in.

Check pet finder or adopt a pet online.

If you have a close friend that is an animal lover, ask them where they found their pet.

I recently adopted a rescued Doberman puppy with my husband and son. Well, I must confess that comparison which compares a baby to a puppy is pretty accurate. My silent hikes under the eucalyptus trees and long walks in the neighborhood have now become dominated by exercising my puppy Fortune. Active, fast and intense, this puppy has brought a new spark into our home. Yes, of course, puppies can be challenging. But the actual act of giving of myself is so satisfying, I feel connected and inspired by dedicating my time and energy to rescuing this puppy. Not to mention the satisfaction of knowing I helped save an animal that might have been euthanized.

I will admit that even though I am a cat person first, I have always loved dogs, too. As a little girl in 4-H Club, I showed my dog Snoopy at the fair in dog obedience training competition. A tragic event happened the night before our dog show. Our dog Puppy which my brother was showing in the competition was hit by a car. Our entire family sat together on the front porch under the stars crying together as we mourned the loss of our family's dog.

Life can be utterly painful. We can lose those that we love or a circumstance of some sort can set us back. Owning a pet and taking care of a pet teaches us lessons in committing our heart, loving something and how to deal with grief. Animals can help our children feel more self-secure and loved which in turn helps build their self-esteem. Losing a pet is not easy. But it also helps us understand the process of life. There are beginnings and ends of chapters with these pets. They will enrich our lives with much love and happiness along the way. I could write another chapter on all of the animals that have filled my soul with joy and love. I could tell you they might just be one of the reasons I turned out to be half as good of a person as I did. Animals are like angels. They give us peace. They give us protection and they make us feel safe always with their love.

The title of this chapter is rescue a pet, but really should be *"rescued by a pet"*, for all they do for us. I am recommending to you that you first check with rescue associations or in the animal shelters to find a pet to fill your life with more love. Remember our journey on our path will be filled with obstacles, tribulations and sometimes hard moments. A pet could just be your one salvation that adds peace and joy to your soul. Anatole France, Nobel Prize winner, once said, *"Until one has loved an animal, a part of one's soul remains unawakened."* Mother Teresa also had wonderful things to say to encourage us to love and protect animals. Her words were:

> *They too are created by the same loving hand of God which Created us… it is our duty to protect them and to promote their well-being.*

So remember these quotes. Remember to nourish your soul by your own action of rescuing a pet in need of a home. After all, your soul is in need of love.

Chapter 14

Dream without Limits

I've always been a dreamer. Ever since I was a little girl I would find a quiet space and make time to allow my mind to envision the grandest details of something in the future. My quiet space just happened to be on the back of my horse, named Patches. His red and white colors marked him like that of one you might see in an old cowboy and Indian movie. I was so proud of my horse Patches. I would ride him bareback when I was growing up in Southern Missouri. My secret quiet space just happened to be in a wide-open field near the corner back fence line under a row of oak trees. After racing across the hayfield as fast as I could ride, Patches and I would rest under the scattered shade and rays of sunlight beaming through the branches and leaves. I was a farm girl. Yes, I ran around barefoot. I rode horses and I lived a sheltered quiet life of a Midwestern girl with an idyllic childhood.

I remember lying back across my horse under the sturdy oak trees, just staring up at the hint of sunlight gleaming with certainty of other places that were awaiting me in my lifetime. I felt certain that however much I loved being a farm girl that I was destined to move to the city. This routine of dreaming under the oak tree carried on for years. These visualizations were so strong and certain there wasn't a doubt in my mind that I would make that happen.

When I graduated from high school back in 1989, I found my way to the nearest city I could find: Kansas City. Next I moved to San Francisco, then New York for a couple of months, and onto Los Angeles. I never had any fear that I was too much of a Midwestern girl; I just knew I belonged there like everyone else. You see all of those years of dreaming under the wide-open space back on the farm on the back of my beloved horse Patches planted a seed of reality that grew a strong vision for my heart to follow.

Now I am looking back over the years and wonder sometimes how I had such confidence to leave my hometown without ever looking back. I must admit that even though I left right out of high school, those hayfields and Midwest values still define who I am on the inside today. I remember my friends from my high school asking me when I would move back to Missouri after I had been in California for a few years. "Never, I am staying here."

They were shocked to say the least. Now I find with age I am dreaming of Missouri. That simple, slow time on the deck during hot summer nights sipping sweet tea, while listening to the frogs singing in the ponds under the moonlight. I still remember the freedom and certainty my dreams built within me at an early age and I know without a doubt that is why I was able to leave so fiercely and independently. I am so thankful for my early dreams that lead me to my current life I am living now. Each choice, each thought soon can materialize in our world. So be careful what you spend your time dwelling on in your mind. You may well receive it one day without warning.

You know that saying, *"Be careful what you wish for…"*

Dream. What exactly does that mean? "A visionary creation of our imagination" is essentially the definition of dreaming. When we take time to use our imagination to experience something we want, we are actively seeking this in our minds. This is in fact an action that you are taking as the first step in making what you want come true. Of course, you must follow up your desire with intense hard work. Struggle will undoubtedly be involved. But isn't it so fun to make what you want come true in the real world? Author and Life Coach Tony Robbins said this about goals, which ties into dreams. He said, "Goals are like magnets. They'll attract the things that make them come true. "

To succeed at a dream or a desire we actively think can benefit our lives also adds to our level of self-confidence and our own personal self-esteem. So if you are one of those pragmatic individuals who think that 'dreaming' is for those that have their head in the clouds, then you need to redefine your idea of what dreaming really means. One of my favorite quotes ever is from the movie *The Bridges of Madison County*:

> *The old dreams were good dreams; they didn't work out, but I'm glad I had them.*

Dreaming allows our mind to take a mental 'time out' from our current reality. By making time to actively seek to build a new idea or next chapter to come in our lives can be very inspiring. Yes, we can't always make all of our wishes come true, but what fun it is to believe in the hope of tomorrow.

I find today's children are so ahead in many ways because of the world of technology. However, there seems to be that missing element of inspiring teenagers to dream big and imagine what they want when they are adults. Too many of us are too busy complaining about the government or unhappy circumstances to pave a way for the imagination to become proactive and start building new dreams to come.

So, yes, I am a middle-aged woman that is no longer a model or an actress. I may be deemed older, more mature. And yes, even be pressured to feel as if I am over the hill.

Time to throw in the towel, right? I don't think so!

Now like no other is your time to discover your gumption in your dreams and to figure out what you want the last half of your life to look like... so take time to define it now. Dream that crazy over the top dream. Believe that it can happen. Be realistic about the steps it will take to achieve it. However, don't settle for less. Don't sell yourself short because you are no longer only eighteen years old.

I now look back and want to thank my younger self for believing in her dreams. I want to thank my younger self for not giving up, not quitting, and for taking time to carve out the world I knew was waiting for me. I may be over forty. I may be that woman that is now targeted with every ad on the planet telling me I need a lift, a tuck, a filler, or eyelash extensions, but I don't let those ads define who I am on the inside. I turn away from their harsh ad campaigns that want me as a woman to feel as if I need help to turn back the hands of time. I urge you, too, to do the same.

Instead, reach inside and build sandcastles to the sky. You might even surprise yourself and accomplish that something special you never thought you could do.

What am I dreaming of right now? Well, I take time each week to dream of moving to Mexico just south of Cancun in a beautiful little town of Playa Del Carmen. I can feel the Caribbean breeze, smell the salty ocean and hear the sound of the tropical birds just outside the home I may some day live in there. I can see the coffee pot percolating as I make toast in the morning. And best of all, I can see my husband's natural smile stay permanently wide because he is living in the place we both feel like is paradise on earth. Wish me luck. I am building sandcastles to the sky... are you? After all, if you don't take time to dream, no one else can do it for you.

Chapter 15

Meditation versus Botox

Meditation. What is it exactly and why would it be related to stopping wrinkles? Did you know that habitual facial expressions used repeatedly over years of time can eventually lead to that indelible wrinkle? "Frown lines between the eyebrows and crow's feet radiating from the corners of the eyes develop as the tiny muscles permanently contract," according to the online source.

If this is so, if we know this in advance, then an easy way to help prevent these creases we so dislike on our face is by becoming cognizant of our moods. Do you know what your facial movements look like when you are using these three particular emotions?

Anger
Sadness
Fear

I ask you now for one week to subject yourself to this test when you can think of it. Pull out a compact mirror to see what you are doing with your muscles on your face during these three powerful emotions. If you can identify when you are frowning and become aware of that movement, you are actively helping fight the battle against wrinkles without spending hundreds of dollars on face fillers that can damage your God-given looks.

I had someone ask me as I was writing this book, "What about someone that has a face that naturally looks like they're frowning. Then what? Are you saying no plastic surgery if you are unhappy with the way your face looks?"

I explained to them, "Yes, actually. That is an important theme in this book. Your natural beauty is something you can work on and change yourself without subjecting yourself to anesthesia." Going under the knife and risking your health is something to seriously investigate before you just haphazardly do so because it seems to be 'trendy' right now. Check out alternative options. Walking into a plastic surgeon's office may seem like the quick fix without much thought involved. But is that really necessary? Ask yourself, could there be a more simplistic approach to modifying your wrinkles?

The answer is… *Yes!*

Remember, your face is the only one you have. So my suggestions are asking you to first do these things:

- Work on your inner self to find more peace, love and joy, which will in turn reflect on your mood, attitude and overall sense of well-being.
- Try alternative methods and products that don't have you placing an X marks the spot on your face with a pen, followed by a needle shooting a substance derived from a poison that can actually kill you. In just the United States, over 3,000 individuals will die from Botulism.
- Take the easy approach. Wear a hat when exposed to the sun too much. Wear sunblock. Take time to actually care and nurture your skin at night. I will address some simple tips in Part Three for you to consider.

Even though the amounts of Botulism will be placed in small doses into your skin, here are some common side effects of Botox:

- Temporary bruising
- Headache
- Respiratory infection
- Flu syndrome
- Drooping of the upper eyelid

- Nausea
- Indigestion
- Losing empathic abilities when communicating with others

Now you might be wondering what this information is doing in the Soul section? This is one more friendly reminder to you to reconsider before you just do the trendy thing. This is a friendly reminder to think beyond skin deep and to reach in to find out why you may be developing the wrinkles you have now. There are ways you can prevent them from becoming worse. How? Relax! Stop being stressed out over your face. Focus inward toward a natural, more peaceful state of mind. This is a reminder to go within yourself first. Seek solace. Unwind that stress you may be carrying daily around in your facial expressions, which can contribute to wrinkles.

Meditation anyone? ZEN time?

If you have time to drive to a plastic surgeon, slap down some money and wait to be poked by a needle, you definitely have time to figure out simple ways to incorporate meditation exercises into your day. Here is a simple meditation assignment that is easy to fit into a hectic schedule.

Lie down on your bed with your head correlating more in a straight line with your spine. Prop your knees up, which will help you with better alignment. (You can use a yoga mat for this, too.) Place your hands together on the base of your stomach. Form a diamond-like shape with your index fingers touching and your thumbs meeting. Your thumbs should be directly below your rib cage. Rest your hands gently on your stomach so you can feel your inhalation and exhalation.

Now focus on taking five deep breaths. Breathe in through your nose and exhale out of your mouth. Make a slight 'Ahh' sound as you release the air. When you are breathing, try to fill the core of your body with as much oxygen as possible. When you do, then hold for a slight moment and release the air slowly, while making the slight 'Ahh' noise. Try to pull your muscles in your stomach all the way to the base of the floor or the mattress on your bed. Then repeat. During this exercise, if you find your mind wandering to something else, redirect your thoughts to your breathing. Observe your breathing and how it feels to your body.

Do this exercise once daily. I usually do this at night before I go to bed. This helps me unlock the worry from my mind. I am fueling my body with healing oxygen, while quietly releasing all of my worries.

One of the fundamental lessons I learned from practicing meditation is that as a society on a whole we tend to be shallow breathers. Our thoughts run at a fast pace racing from moment to moment. When we take a cognitive moment to intake a full deep breath, we can shift our minds and help return our energy inside our bodies, giving us a more grounded feeling. Always try to stay rooted in your body. What does that mean exactly? Well think of a tree and how their roots grow deep within the earth's soil. Imagine your feet rooted to the ground below you throughout the day so you are more present. Keeping our energy and our thoughts directed inward to our breath helps keep us more relaxed and even-keeled.

Just recently I had an overwhelming week ahead of me. I wasn't quite sure how I would manage so much extra multi-tasking on top of my current schedule. For over half of that day I had a slight headache. I tried to process how I could make this week go by faster because I knew it would be hectic. My nerves were shot and I felt irritable.

I know from my own experience with practicing meditation that this can be changed. I can return to my breath and help calm my mind. Although life can simply take our minds somewhere else, we sometimes forget what we know. At the end of the evening that day, I laid in bed looking up at the ceiling... and I remembered my meditation exercise. I propped my knees up, and laid my hands on my stomach in the diamond-like position. I took five deep breaths. After I finished, I added some visualization of how I wanted each day to go. I poured loving thoughts on this hectic week. I imagined each day going perfectly and smoothly. I did the exercise again, and finally drifted off into a peaceful sleep.

Many of us think of meditation as a 45-minute ordeal that has us sitting on the floor in a spaghetti-like position. What I learned when I studied meditation is that the quieting of the mind is returning your breath. Even if it's one deep, mindful breath that returns you to your center.

At the back of the book I have some suggested reading, which includes *Mental Fitness,* by Michiko. This book is laid out in simple terms with many meditation and visualization exercises that are easy to understand and do.

So remember before you take time out of your life to fill your face with a foreign substance that does not belong there naturally, make an active choice to go deeper first. Work on your mind, body and soul. You might be surprised at what you uncover when you only take a few moments to look within your soulful self each night before you turn out the lights.

Part Two – Your Health

The only time to eat diet food is while you're waiting for the steak to cook.

~ Julia Child

Chapter 16

Your Health

Being a model at a young age had its advantages and disadvantages. Imagine constantly weighing in and measuring yourself because if you don't you might lose out on that income to pay the bills. Imagine standing in line next to hordes of beautiful young girls thinner, taller, sexier and maybe even more beautiful than you. Those were the beginning chapters that founded my youth. While my friends were hitting the tanning beds and perming their hair every six months, I had an agent that said no to perms and to tanning beds. No to certain foods and yes to looking healthy for the next photo shoot. I happened to be a teenager during the late 80s, which meant that a size four–six was considered beautiful, and being a skeleton stick then was out. Curves were in then: Christie Brinkley, Paulina Porizkova and Cindy Crawford. These women were my point of reference on beauty as a teenager. So when I say thin, I'm not speaking of what we associate nowadays with young models. A recent study showed that supermodels today compared with supermodels in the early 90s are 23% thinner. In this very important section of the beauty trinity, I will share one interview with a doctor that lists the healthy weight size for your frame.

So my idea of looking healthy is not being super thin, while being married to the best plastic surgeon in town. I am no one's creation except my own. Health is not about being thin. Health is about how you take care of the physical body and what you put into it. It's not a gluten-free craze. It's not organic either. Your health is individually different from the next person. My suggestions here in this all-important part of the beauty trinity have worked for many and can work for you, too. I am going to share with you simple supplements, a healthy lifestyle diet, plus a workout routine that does not have you spending two hours at the gym. Health is about taking proper care of your body that in turn aligns with your soul and beauty. If your health is lacking, your soul will suffer, as well as your natural beauty. Health is not about yo-yo diets, eating only apples and slapping off the buns to hamburgers. The Julia Child quote, *"The only time to eat diet food is while you are waiting for the steak to cook,"* happens to capture how most of us feel when we hear the word 'diet' being forced into our lives.

Julia Child might not have been a health nut but she made women feel French in America as they learned to debone a duck effortlessly, while inspiring women and men around the world to cook amazing food. The point here is real food counts.

So you say you may be a vegan. You might be a vegetarian. Maybe you are a fruitatarian that only eats what falls from trees and you don't cook it because you are killing a vegetable.

That's okay, here, too. I am suggesting you throw away diet fads for real food. I am going to suggest to you one diet that is more of a lifestyle based on results, delicious food that has you counting down to less than twenty days on the calendar. This does not include milkshakes, or prepackaged meals. If you can learn how to change your lifestyle with better nutrition, not only will you feel and look better, you will also lose weight, too. The best news is the results happen… *fast!*

Albert Einstein once said regarding health:

> *The devil has put a penalty on all things we enjoy in life. Either we suffer in health or we suffer in soul or we get fat.*

My question is to you as a reader, do you believe that statement? If you do, then you are limiting yourself to a small box with less opportunity of success of feeling good and optimum health. We are what our thoughts are. So if you can actively seek to place your health at the top of your MOST IMPORTANT 'TO-DO' list then you can prove that quote as being misguided. During my mid-thirties I had to seek help to learn how to start eating healthier. What I learned is that there was no suffering involved in feeling and looking great.

Why does one have to suffer? If you can find the tools to work on your mental health and outer appearance as a daily practice in your weekly routine, there is no reason for the other 'shoe to drop'.

The choice is yours. The question is, are you going to choose _you_ before you choose your food?

Do know though some effort might be involved here for you. You may have to change what you eat in order to feel better daily. You might have to consciously make a strenuous effort to improve your mental attitude in order to improve your health. While obesity is on the rise in America, it's never been more important to actively seek a healthier lifestyle by making YOURSELF a priority.

I will share my interviews with three doctors and a nutritionist that share their knowledge, attitude and inside research that has proven the results you may be searching for right now during your midlife phase.

In this section I will be revealing these life-changing Health choices that can help improve your well-being.

- A life-giving molecule that combats aging, boosts your immune system and improves your mood.
- A vinegar that can improve your daily health, fight weight gain and stabilize your blood sugar.
- A key supplement that can affect and improve your brain function, combat weight gain, and improve your skin.
- A lifestyle choice from one diet that can actually work! I will list the source with a fantastic one on one interview with the _New York Times_ Bestselling author Dr. Mike

Moreno.
- Why the philosophy behind 15 minutes or less can affect your waistline.
- Find out which needle injection is a must and it has nothing to do with wrinkles.
- Sophistication versus health: which will you choose?
- Food tips that are delicious, and drinks to discard and replace with the right drink.

I also interview some outstanding other experts as well. As a woman over forty, I feel fantastic. Why? Due to my lifestyle changes and choices I have actively applied each day for many years. With the early beginnings in my career focused on weight and size, I discovered why our 'lifestyle' choices affect our appearance. In these next few chapters I reveal these small active choices that have literally changed my health, happiness and mood.

I will also share with you moments where I have experienced unwanted weight gain. I will reveal to you how I shaved off those pounds, which didn't involve hours of exercise or crazy diet fads. I now feel better at the age of 41 than I did when I was 25. The years do keep ticking by… the question is for all of us to decide, which path will you take? Like Health Guru Dr. Patricia Bragg posed the question in one of her books: *"Are you on the road to health and longevity or sickness and disease?"* After all, you only have one body. You better take care of it!

Chapter 17

Life Giving Molecule: Melatonin

There just happens to be this amazing little secondhand bookshop in the town of Rancho Santa Fe, California called 'The Book Cellar'. Due to my overwhelming love of reading and my dislike of reading by way of technology, you could say discovering this wonderful bookstore felt like I had discovered some secret treasure trove I could visit for a moment of joy for my weekly routine. Imagine a small, neatly kept little shop of books with a little red awning above the door, with recent titles on all topics existing inside the tranquility and silence adjacent to the main library in town. Usually, I would browse for my favorite authors, which range from Luanne Rice and Alice Hoffman in America, to Maeve Binchy and Kate Kerrigan in Ireland. I went through a phase where I read every Maeve Binchy, then to reading five consecutive Alice Hoffman novels in one sitting. Reading happens to be one of my soulful 'joys' that allows me to connect within myself, find peace and nourish that important part of the beauty trinity. However, I had no idea that it would lead to a major discovery that has contributed to one of the most important health discoveries during my middle-aged years.

In the health and wellness section, I happened to notice a book with a bold blue banner in white font that read *Melatonin* by Russel J. Reiter, Ph.D. and Jo Robinson.

Underneath the title read these four important factors:
- Combat Aging
- Boost Your Immune System
- Reduce Your Risk of Cancer and Heart Disease
- Get a Better Night's Sleep

Now I know what you are thinking. That's why I picked up this book to read it. That would seem to be the obvious thought here because those four things mentioned are quite remarkable! However, just like you and most of the world, I thought melatonin was just an over-the-counter pill that helped me sleep better at night.

Well, that's what I thought before I stopped taking melatonin every day. The backstory on why I bought this book and broke out of my fiction craze is because I had just discovered melatonin that year. (I know, it's been around for awhile. I'm a little late in the game, but you know what they say… better late than…) I started taking it because my husband had a bottle in the medicine cabinet. Well after a few restless nights, I started taking melatonin daily. Well, guess what? I felt great. I had not linked it to melatonin yet because I only realized that fact after I stopped taking it daily. I recognized my mood, attitude and overall state of well-being felt more aligned and improved. So I bought my own first bottle of melatonin. The only problem was I didn't really have a clue why it affected my entire day versus just my sleeping patterns. I had thought melatonin was just for sleeping… *Wrong.*

Yes, melatonin does help you sleep more deeply and soundly. But on that day as I stood in my favorite bookstore staring at the bold blue banner proclaiming melatonin's miracle secrets, I knew this book would answer my questions.

I opened the *Melatonin* book to the table of contents and read these headings:
- Meet Melatonin: What does it do for you?
- The Best Antioxidant: Unsurpassed protection against dangerous free radicals
- A Master Sex Hormone
- Boosting the Immune System

These were just a few of the headlines that had my jaw dropping as my mouth formed that perfect 'O' shape with that feeling of knowing you are about to discover some incredible secret that will change your life.

I know what you are thinking here. Really? Melatonin? Isn't that for sleeping?

No. Well, yes, but no. Melatonin does so much more. Let's just say I was incredibly inspired by this newfound information inside Dr. RJ Reiter and Jo Robinson's book that unlocked the *why* of this well-known supplement. I began taking the book with me everywhere. I called my parents daily and begged them to start taking melatonin daily. I am not normally a bully. But during this craze for me over melatonin, I was.

"Mom, are you taking your melatonin?"

Silence.

"Well, you need to run out and buy it immediately. Don't you want to feel better today and live an extra ten years?"

"Yes, Machel (sounds like Michelle) we do," my mom would respond. I even wrapped it up in Christmas wrapping paper for my parents to have this book at their fingertips. I felt like this news *I had to share* because it had so radically changed the way I felt each day. You can imagine my delight as I opened her medicine cabinet to see her little bottle nestled next to the skin creams.

Why did taking Melatonin improve my health so much? Well, here are some simple facts:

Melatonin is a natural hormone created by the pineal gland in the center of our brain. This is a natural hormone we produce that plays a vital role with our cells. According to Dr. Reiter's research, "Death occurs when we have lost a significant number of vital cells." This hormone and antioxidant helps aid our body in fighting off diseases and toxins. With age this all-important hormone declines.

Which is where I enter onto the scene as a middle-aged woman that's suddenly feeling fabulous again after taking melatonin. Who knew that this supplement was a hormone we naturally created in our brain? I didn't. If I had learned that back in biology many eons ago... let's just say at that age melatonin didn't sound that exciting to a teenager. So yes, if you are paying attention, the reason why we need to take melatonin now is because our body actually needs to supplement our natural loss of this hormone known to combat cancer, lower blood pressure, diabetes and, last but not least, sleep better at night.

Maybe I had an unusually low amount of melatonin. All I can tell you is for six months I kept spouting facts and figures to my parents and to all of my friends. One of my friends replied:

"Oh, I sleep fine."

Melatonin is not just about sleep. This has to do with learning the facts, applying what you know and enhancing your health with knowledge already out there for you to discover at the fingertips. There is a reason why this chapter is the first one in the Health section. I know from the bottom of my toes hitting the pavement that if I stop taking my melatonin supplement, my immune system, overall sense of well-being and mood will begin to decline. Some like prescription drugs. I happen to stick with melatonin. Just make sure you take it two hours before you go to bed.

I also suggest you read the label when you go to the pharmacy and pick up your own bottle of melatonin now. Make sure that you just buy one with only melatonin. Three to five milligrams is perfect for me but see what works best for you. I use Nature Made brand.

Before I end on this note, one of the most exciting events that occurred, Dr. RJ Reiter was kind enough to allow me to interview him for this important chapter on Health in the Beauty Trinity. I asked him three important questions, plus his permission to share facts from the book that began a new beginning for me –

life after melatonin.

And in case you are wondering, there are no side effects. Yes, if you want to just use this for a sleep aid, that is just one of the many benefits of melatonin.

Here is my interview with Dr. Reiter:

What led you to devote so much of your life to the research of melatonin?

Dr. Reiter: I began research on melatonin when I was a captain in the Medical Service Corps at Edgewood Arsenal, MD. This molecule had only recently been discovered, and we were investigating its potential use in the space program. At that time I got 'hooked' on melatonin because of the remarkable actions it has. Even today, I believe we are only seeing the 'tip of this iceberg'.

Besides sleeping, what other benefits can melatonin do for women and men over the age of forty?

Dr. Reiter: Sleep promotion is only one of many actions it has. Importantly, it aids in the regulation of biological rhythmicity, which is important for optimal health. To do this, it acts on the biological clock in the brain. Additionally, melatonin is a powerful antioxidant and protects all cells against damage from free radicals. This relates to many maladies since free radical damage contributes to many disease processes, particularly later in life. Examples include: atherosclerosis, dementia, skin deterioration, hyperglycemia, inflammation, cataracts etc, etc.

I have noticed a significant change in my skin since I started taking melatonin two years ago. How does melatonin work toward anti-aging?

Dr. Reiter: The beneficial actions on the skin relate to the antioxidant activity of melatonin. Skin damage, e.g. crow's feet, is a result of free radical damage. There are already many skin creams available that contain the antioxidant melatonin.

So what are you going to do tomorrow? Run out to a pharmacy and buy melatonin. Especially if you are over the age of forty. Go buy it today. Thank you, Dr. Reiter, for devoting your life to helping others discover this amazing hormone in a pill form to help us age with more vitality, zest and vigor.

Three things to remember:

You lose your natural melatonin as you age, which helps aid your body in proper sleep and fighting off disease.

Melatonin is a natural anti-aging hormone.

Melatonin helps build up your immune system. So buy a bottle today!

Chapter 18

Apple Cider Vinegar: Nature's Healing Miracle

During my mid-thirties I used to frequent this fun hip health store that just made you feel good about yourself because you were buying your food there. You know the kind. There is a counter in the store with an employee wearing a string of white beads around their neck and a green apron as they proudly take orders to make every kind of vegetable juice concoction right in front of your eyes. You can buy vegetarian lunchmeat in thin slices if you happen to disdain 'real meat'. There is an arrangement of nuts lined up in plastic shoot containers that you can bag yourself. Just weigh the nuts at the checkout counter. There may even be little food samples in the vegetable aisles from organic citrus to freshly made salsa with a bag of organic tortilla chips.

This health food store became one of my little joys that I rewarded myself with during a busy workweek. That's when I made one of the most important health discoveries of my life: apple cider vinegar. I will start out by letting you know that I might not have made this important discovery without the free sample. After hearing some important factors from the employee that day, I made my first purchase of Bragg's Apple Cider Vinegar.

I began to religiously keep one bottle in my refrigerator every week. I would drink just about two tablespoons in the morning and in the evening when I remembered to take it. I still can remember the first week I began taking it; I am not exaggerating when I say I felt like 'superwoman'. My life sprang into action. Not only did I feel more energetic, I had more mental clarity and sharpness than my life prior to Bragg Apple Cider Vinegar. I remember expressing joy and enthusiasm to my inner circle regarding this new discovery. And just like melatonin I wasn't sure why this affected my health with such positive effects. I just knew the results were *real*. Soon I began to read online and in bookstores why ACV invigoratingly rejuvenated overall mood. I found out that Hippocrates in 400 BC had used this to treat his patients. He is known as the Father of Medicine – using ACV to treat his patients like we use antibiotics today to fight off germs and much more.

Here are some more important facts that you need to know about Apple Cider Vinegar and why you should add this to your list. These facts are from Patricia Bragg's book *Apple Cider Vinegar: Miracle Health System*:

- Helps promote a youthful skin and vibrant body.
- Helps control and normalize body weight.
- Helps digestion, assimilation and helps balance the pH.
- Helps fight viruses, bacteria, and mold naturally.
- Helps detox the body so sinus, asthma and flu sufferers can breathe easier and more normally.
- Helps retard old age onset in humans and pets.
- Helps regulate calcium metabolism.
- Helps fight arthritis.
- Helps banish acne.
- Helps fight diabetes.

(Please read this book by Dr. Patricia Bragg if you would like to find out more scientific evidence behind the benefits of apple cider vinegar.)

Now this list is just endless on the power of natural ACV. When I found out more information, I began to understand why I felt such an incredible difference when I took ACV. From speeding up my daily metabolism to stabilizing my blood sugar I can attest that this is one of the most important recommendations I am suggesting to you in my book *Middle Age Beauty*. I hope you don't confuse this with regular vinegar. And if you are wondering does it have to be Bragg brand, I personally don't recommend other brands and can tell a significant difference in the taste and overall effect it has on my body; Bragg is the best. You can order it directly from them or find it in health food stores. But don't just take my advice. Try it yourself. Incorporate it into your daily routine. I don't leave the house without my two morning tablespoons. I can tell you when I run out and I have gone a few days without ACV, I immediately notice the difference. When I tell you I am sprinting to the health food store for my weekly bottle this is not an exaggeration.

Why? Knowledge is power. Every other product you see in the health food stores are following behind the Bragg's original ACV line. So why not buy the best? In my pursuit of Middle Age Beauty, I passionately pursued obtaining an interview with Dr. Patricia Bragg who is known and respected worldwide for implementing, empowering and teaching others important health secrets besides just taking Apple Cider Vinegar. After four months of contacting the Bragg company, you can imaging my elated, smiling face when I found out that Patricia Bragg would indeed let me interview her for this important chapter in my Health section. (Remember to always ask again in a new way if it's something you are really after!)

Patricia Bragg's vibrant and enthusiastic spirit has inspired millions. Her personal crusade has personally affected my life in such a positive light that this chapter is crucial to your health as well.

Here is my one on one interview with Dr. Patricia Bragg:

Patricia, why is it so important for those in their middle ages to add Apple Cider Vinegar to their diets every day?'

Patricia Bragg: Apple Cider Vinegar is the miracle health system in keeping the body healthy. Hippocrates the 'Father of

Medicine' in 400 BC treated his patients with amazing raw apple cider vinegar because he recognized the powerful cleansing and healing properties. It's a natural occurring antibiotic and natural antiseptic. It fights germs, viruses, bacteria and even mold. There are many internal benefits – it is rich in miracle enzymes and potassium, it improves digestion and assimilation. People with GERDS can sip ½ teaspoon before mealtime. It relieves sore throats and laryngitis, and helps remove toxins and cholesterol.

How do you recommend those, that feel it's hard to swallow naturally, drink apple cider vinegar? Is there a certain way that you think is best? If so why?

Patricia Bragg: Natural, organic, raw apple cider vinegar is a miracle. You can slowly get used to it by taking a teaspoon of the vinegar in 6 oz of purified water. If you desire a sweet taste, you may add some raw honey. Here is the way I suggest: 1–2 teaspoons vinegar with 1–2 teaspoons raw honey into an 8 oz glass of purified or distilled water.

Here is the Bragg's Apple Cider Vinegar Cocktail:

1–2 teaspoons Bragg's Organic Apple Cider Vinegar
1–2 teaspoons of raw honey, agave nectar or pure maple syrup (optional, to taste)
8 ounces purified or distilled water
Note: If diabetic, use 2 Stevia herbal drops

Do you think apple cider vinegar can help weight loss? If so, how and why?

Patricia Bragg: Millions are searching for more natural ways to lose unwanted pounds. Apple cider vinegar is getting results. The pectin found in apples is one of the benefits attributed to the correlation between apple cider vinegar and weight loss. Pectin, a natural fiber, helps clean out the digestive tract; plus, the acidic nature of apple cider vinegar helps stimulate a bodily response that burns stored fat which accelerates weight loss. Dr. Ann

Louise Gittleman, in her book, *The Fat Flush Plan*, uses Bragg's Apple Cider Vinegar as a prime ingredient for seasoning and cooking foods. She found that blood sugar becomes normalized so that people can digest their foods and proteins so much more effectively when using the Bragg's Organic Apple Cider Vinegar. It's perfect for salads, greens, and especially for making the delicious Bragg's Vinegar Cocktail.

I drink 16 ounces a week myself. I have noticed I overall feel better and I hardly ever have colds now. Does apple cider vinegar help improve your immune system as well? Do you find that it is more important for those in their middle ages to take more precautions and better care of themselves?

Patricia Bragg: Yes, it helps keep the immune system in top force! I feel that each person should take charge of their own health, especially after the age of 18. You are what you eat, drink, breathe, think, say, and do.

What do you feel is the biggest mistake those in their middle ages make when it comes to their diet? Yo-yo dieting? Not enough sleep? Too much alcohol intake? If you could recommend they stop one thing to improve their health what would it be?

Patricia Bragg: I feel that people should become their own health captain. They need to realize that what they put in their mouth is fuel, and it can bring either health or sickness. It's up to them to safeguard what they put into their body. It's a prudent fact that they took a group of seniors in their 80s and 90s and fed them a healthy lifestyle (including exercise and weight training!). They all became healthier and felt younger.

You look absolutely amazing. How have you kept your zest, beauty and youthful spirit over the years? If you had one inside secret to share with someone feeling insecure about their middle-aged era, what secret would you share?

Patricia Bragg: I say to all women over 40, 50, 60 – forget the calendar years! If you start worrying about the years as they roll by, whooo, it'll make you old. I feel like I'm 18. I do my exercises every day, I fast for 24 hours, one day a week, on 8 glasses of purified water (with 2 teaspoons of Bragg's Apple Cider Vinegar in 3 of these glasses). I do this for internal cleansing, as it keeps me young. I've never been obese. Your waistline is your lifeline and dateline: the bigger the waistline the shorter the lifespan! Before I put food in my mouth that goes into my stomach tank, I ask, "Is this something that's going to bring me health, energy and beauty? Year after year I'd go to my class reunion; I'd give out Bragg Health and Fitness Books to my school friends. I'm sad to report that now over half of them have demised. The ones that are left are not doing very well: hip and knee replacements, all sorts of major operations, some hard of hearing, poor eyesight, poor posture, and many obese. Why? WHY??? It's because they didn't take charge of their own bodies' health.

The key in life is to take measures that can help us optimize our day to our best performance. Incorporating ACV into my diet has been one extra choice that adds bounce, clarity and an overall positive day for me. So do take my advice here and buy some today. When I run out and skip a few days, I can tell a noticeable difference. So don't skip out! I just wish I had made this discovery sooner. Thank you, Patricia, for the interview. I know you are a wonderful role model to many. Remember, take the little measures like this that don't break your wallet which can literally improve your daily health and mood.

Chapter 19

Take Swimsuit Pictures Once a Year

Yes. That's right. You need to find that little bikini that you are willing to allow yourself to be photographed in by your husband, friend or loved one. I started doing this three years ago with my husband and it absolutely works wonders. Why? Because this involves shedding clothes and seeing what you really look like in front of a camera. And listen, you don't have to be a size four to do this. The goal though for most of the year is to watch what you eat, and do take time to find a routine with working out and stick to it.

This helps me do my extra sit-ups in the morning. This encourages me to walk that extra loop around my block when I may just really want to eat frozen yogurt. This is a visual that propels me forward each year with the thought, "Wow, not bad for 39... Wow, not bad for forty... Wow, not bad for 41..." and so on. Visuals work well with children. Visuals work well with teenagers. Visuals work well with adults. It may sound sort of silly to write that, but if you want to feel glamorous and beautiful how can you do that if you don't have any images to inspire you to keep looking good?

To some of you this may sound shallow. *"Oh, yes, let's be photographed in a bikini and that will make me feel healthy."* Well, what you put in your mouth and what you do with your weight will definitely be influenced once you do your bikini shots once a year. The swimsuit does not have to be a two-piece. Go for conservative if you aren't quite comfortable baring it all in your photos, even if it's just for yourself. This visual of you in a bikini though will motivate you like nothing else.

Just when you want to grab that tub of buttery popcorn at the movie theatre, think back to the bikini picture that solidifies, "I feel great about my body! Look at me."

We may all not get to be Raquel Welch in a poster, but why not try for yourself? The photo shoot with my husband is always so much fun. We don't use any fancy camera. We don't bring any props or lights. We just find a secluded destination where I can feel comfortable to relax, smile and have some fun.

Of course, if you need to diet first and lose some weight, this could be the peak of the mountain that you are aiming for at the end of the year. You can climb it, achieve it and then have forever bikini shots that don't let you forget, "Hey, I like this body. I have a beautiful body." So many women are at odds with their body, their weight and their self-image. The most important step first is to love ourselves inward to out, placing our self-esteem, our confidence into action so we are motivated to do the rest. If you feel depressed, if you feel insecure, the last thing you are going to want to do is wear a bikini in a photo. This is why the "Soul" section is number one. Align your spirit by nourishing your mind and centering your thoughts to positive information. Only speak softly and be positive about yourself. Never put yourself down to anyone. Why? Because people usually believe what you tell them. If you tell someone you have an issue or you are feeling vulnerable, that will be their view of you. So toughen up on the inside first. See yourself successful in your daily life with your friends and family and the rest will start to follow. That's right. The diet, the working out, your attitude will shine and others will see it, too.

This is one tiny motivator that has added much fun and excitement to the last three years of my life. Women need to have a self-positive image of themselves that they can hold in their hand as a testament that, yes, I may be in my middle age period in my life, but darn I look good.

So you are a few pounds heavier than where you should be, now is the time to do something about it. One of the fastest things that can age us and worse – send us into a state of feeling lethargic and tired – is carrying around more weight than our body frame should.

So this chapter is the precursor, the prequel to you beginning to check in with how you can feel and look the absolute best about yourself *now*. Set a goal with that special someone and get to work. Join a gym. Hit a hiking trail. Walk laps in your neighborhood. Get moving and take action on the very most important person in the world to you – yourself. Reread Patricia Bragg's words of encouragement. There is no reason why aging means we are 'put out to pasture' as an animal like a wild cougar or someone that lacks the zest of a 25 year old.

Get ready to find out how you are going to be bikini ready for your photo shoot so you can reach for the stars and love your body and love your natural self.

How to Prepare for the Swimsuit photo shoot:

- You will need to moderate your diet and learn what foods will help you slim down, while skipping the protein shakes at the grocery store. Next chapter I will share with you an interview from one doctor that has gained worldwide attention for his amazing health plan that is easy to do and incorporate into your everyday life.
- You will need to start working out weekly and sticking to your commitment to yourself. You will need to visualize the body you are aiming for. Hold that mental picture and remind yourself that you have a goal you are working toward that will reward you with tangible proof you can hold in your hands.
- You will need to stop making excuses because of your age, your busy schedule and where you live. I will be introducing some simple things that you can do for exercise in your home if you can't find time to make it to a gym.
- Find one friend to make the commitment with you. Choose a date and make the commitment together. This will be fun, too.

Also, you will find out in one of my next chapters what you must say goodbye to, to help shrink that midriff for that fun bikini shoot only three to six months away. Remember to dream without limits. So dare to imagine the body you want if you aren't quite there, yet. Set your goal and now get going. Trust me the reward of having your photo taken once a year, each year, of what you look like in a bathing suit at your best is a strong mental image to help you with your willpower against eating fast food, buttery popcorn, sugary colas and candy. This picture will motivate you to return to your health conscious ways. Remember, we need to motivate ourselves to be and look our best. To take pride in our body is actually a marvelous feeling.

If we don't set goals like this for ourselves no one will. So let's find out now how to get bikini ready for that photo you can only share with yourself; or post it to your Facebook profile with much pride and accomplishment. Dare to be about 'me'. I don't mean don't be humble or forget others. I mean make yourself your own priority by taking care of you first. Watch the world make more sense and the tension ease off as you begin to discover your most dynamic self is awesome.

Chapter 20

Weigh In with Yourself

During my mid-thirties I met the man of my dreams. We had so much fun when we first started dating. We went to dinners. We had cocktail hours. We hosted intimate parties for our closest friends. This fun, love and good parties I must say were some of the most memorable times of my life. After living in Hollywood, who knew that so many good times were still ahead of me in the sleepy town of Rancho Santa Fe? This affluent community is also where I write my own social column that highlights the local residents. This period of my life felt like my own version of single girls looking for love, except without the skyscrapers and expensive shoe shopping. This extravagant lifestyle of eating out and fun cocktails eventually added up in many pounds on the scale.

However, I was in complete denial about it. I had no idea what my weight was and continued on this path until I began to march closer to my wedding date. Yes, that one dress. Those photos, that last a lifetime, to your soul mate. Now this is where I come clean. I am going to tell you the inside story that is rather embarrassing. Because of my column, I had gained the attention of a local doctor that contacted me to do his weight loss program.

Yes, that's right…weigh loss program. I was absolutely mortified. I went into his office and realized that if I accepted I would soon be weighing in and participating in a rather humili-ating experience (so I thought at that point in my life because of my previous years as a model). Well, guess what? I eventually accepted. I weighed in with reality. Guess how much weight I had gained after fifteen months of blissful love?

Thirty-five pounds.

Yes, that's right. I am confessing to you that weight gain is very easy. Especially if you are over thirty and not eating a smart or a healthy diet. I managed to swallow my pride, take some advice and counseling on nutrition from a doctor. Guess what happened? I lost the weight, all of my weight, in less than four months. What I have not mentioned yet is that I did continue to work out consistently during those fifteen months of weight gain. I had been eating more fast foods with my younger husband, who can eat anything and not gain a pound; I assumed I could, too...

Wrong!

The good news is I lost 25 of that prior to my wedding date and another ten before my honeymoon. I was actually able to fit back into my bikini again and wear it with confidence. This is when I began to make my swimsuit photos part of my yearly goal to keep me in shape and on my toes.

One of the first things I had to give up in order to participate in this diet that helped me shed those pounds was... alcohol. This period back in 2009 shifted my health in the most positive place for the rest of my life. Not only did I lose weight, but I became educated on my diet, what to eat and what not to eat for a woman that was no longer naturally thin without trying. Now I don't really diet. Out of all of the diets on the market today, what resembles the diet I did that year comes from another doctor in San Diego. Dr. Mike Moreno.

Dr. Moreno practices here in San Diego. He also works with a lot of patients that have diabetes and need to lose weight. Due to his active health conscious and caring nature as a doctor, he wrote a book that is now known as *The 17 Day Diet* which quickly became a *New York Times* Bestseller. You can imagine how thrilled I was when Dr. Moreno seemed genuinely excited to be interviewed for my book.

Before I share his interview with you I want to urge you to check in with your weight. When was the last time you weighed yourself? Have you gained some extra pounds but are afraid to admit it just like I was with my own weight? That's okay. Never fear. The best news is like anything, this journey into eating right and exercising more can be fun, exhilarating and just what you need to feel better about yourself.

Weight is one of the most important factors that can cause us to age prematurely. So keeping off those extra pounds during our middle age years are important for so many factors. What is my main motivator to stay in shape? I am just a happier person when I can fit into my skinny jeans! Who doesn't want to feel happy, right?

Back to Dr. Moreno and his amazing diet that feels more like a lifestyle choice because you can actually eat! Dr. Moreno also explains in health terms the importance of why your weight management is so important for your health. His book doesn't only tell you what to eat, but how to incorporate this new lifestyle by offering you recipes and meal plans that are easy to follow. One of his number one rules is to try not to eat out, and buy your groceries and cook at home. As I have already confessed to you my weight gain nightmare of 35 pounds, do yourself a favor and think about *yourself* first before you choose your food.

Here is a man that is inspiring to many, including my parents! My dad has lost over fifty pounds on the 17 Day Diet. Not only did my parents lose weight, they became inspired, and enjoy their new eating habits. They do not feel like they are even dieting. That's why this is my recommendation to you. Learn about food and how to eat properly. Plan your meals and choose a healthy lifestyle over gluttony and self-indulgence.

Here is my interview with *New York Times* Bestselling author, Dr. Mike Moreno:

In your book *The 17 Day Diet* you encourage your readers to walk 17 minutes a day, once in the morning and once in the evening. That seems easy enough. Do you find that making

time for exercise tends to be a stumbling block for many? And if so, what advice would you give to someone that feels blocked on 'making' time when they are already so busy in their daily schedule?

Dr. Mike: Yes. I think that a lot of people use their busy lives as an excuse to not exercise. I know times are tough and there are many that are working two to three different jobs. I try to get my patients to focus on what they CAN do.

Never underestimate your efforts. Never feel like any little bit of effort or progress isn't meaningful. Anything you can do and progress you can make, whether in exercise or your efforts in diet, is REALLY valuable in making progress. If walking 30 minutes a day is tough on you, then walk six minutes five times a day or even three minutes 10 times a day. You will get there. It will get easier, and try not to be so hard on yourself. If you lost a pound this week and your goal was two pounds, you can achieve your goal. Focus on what you CAN do, not on what you can't do, and that can help you overcome your block toward exercising.

My parents are both on your 17 Day Diet plan right now. They enjoy the meal suggestions that you share in your book. Do you find that the success of your 17 Day Diet plan has been because it's 'less' like a diet and more like a lifestyle choice?

Dr. Mike: Yes. In order for any successful weight loss, 'long-term' can feel insurmountable in the beginning. Making time and outlining your week and your meals can become an easy and exciting lifestyle that anyone can incorporate into their daily schedule. The book gives many examples with creative breakfast, lunch and dinner choices which keep that 17 day diet fun and enjoyable, while making immediate progress in terms of losing weight and feeling healthier in a short amount of time.

Your diet is done in four simple cycles of 17 days. This number seems attainable. What kinds of immediate shifts and changes can someone expect from experiencing the first 17 days?

Dr. Mike: Immediate. Someone that has never tried my diet before can expect changes within five to seven days. That includes feeling healthier and having more energy as well as losing weight immediately in the first few days. Their mood and overall sense of well-being will improve, too. Most of my patients become enthusiastic by the immediate results. With each small achievement, you will feel empowered to make this important transition with your lifestyle and your diet.

What originally motivated you to develop the 17 Day Diet Plan? As a physician living in San Diego, you launched "Walk with Your Doc", in which you still participate with your patients every week. How rewarding is that for you to know that your diet and your walking program have helped enrich and empower so many that have struggled with their weight?

Dr. Mike: The first part to the answer would be my diabetic patients. I based the 17 day diet plan on a similar plan that I saw rapid success with for my diabetic patients in San Diego. I launched "Walk with Your Doc" when one of my patients lost their walking partner. She said her walking partner had moved. So I volunteered to walk with her on Tuesdays and Thursdays. The nurses sent out a flyer and a group formed. We have over fifty to sixty people walking. As a doctor that cares so much for his patients, it very rewarding to see the impact and success for them, just like those that do the 17 Day Diet program.

What parting words of encouragement could you add that might inspire someone who has never really tried to manage their weight and health as a reason to start now?

Dr. Mike: We are never too old or too young to start taking care of ourselves NOW. If you make the effort to change, your body will reward you by feeling better right away. Make time to do the 17-minute workout twice a day, even if you have to split up your time. Move out of your comfort zone and you'll start to accomplish things you've only dreamed of… you won't regret it.

The day I interviewed Dr. Mike was like one of those days that stand out, when life feels like it makes perfect sense when we apply ourselves to do better, learn and care about ourselves as our number one priority. His book is always handy in my house. One of my favorite recipes is an eggplant parmesan dish that tastes like you are dining out for the night! Also take Julia Child's advice. She said, "Learn how to cook – try new recipes, learn from your mistakes, be fearless and above all have fun!" You can apply this to your approach to managing and losing weight.

You have one body. You have one life.

Do your best to stay in check with your weight. Have fun in planning your meals. Be realistic about a weight you can maintain. Remember when you think thin, think back to the 80s when the Super Models actually had some curves to their bodies. Remember your weight is something you need to be honest with yourself about. So buy a scale and weigh in at least once a month. We can't all be super models but we can shoot for a healthy weight that makes us feel great about the way we look and feel every day. Why not dare to wiggle into a pair of your favorite skinny jeans? I do. After all, you only have one body! Don't let your age be the excuse of your extra weigh anymore. Do something about it. Take action and rethink your food, your lifestyle and make yourself your number one priority.

Some key factors to remember why this diet is right for you:

- 4 easy cycles of seventeen days.
- This diet encourages you to eat 'real foods' with simple recipes that are easy to prepare at home.
- You can eat fruit!
- When you reach one point of the cycle you can take breaks and eat what you want on the weekend.
- Based on eating natural foods, no premade dinners or

milkshakes.

- Promotes eating properly for your Glycemic level, which helps keep diabetes at bay.

This is a choice of lifestyle really, NOT a diet.

Remember that your weight is truly an important part of your health equation and so is your diet. So do monitor what you eat. Do be mindful of your food and always think about yourself first before you make that next meal choice. After all, you only have one body; why not look and feel fabulous, too?

Chapter 21

Easy Diet Tips and Food Suggestions That Can Help You Manage Your Weight

My husband manages and operates his family's business that just happens to be a classic produce and gift shop. Yes, do think upscale modernized fruit stand. Becoming my husband's wife also meant benefiting from helping run this business that's based on selling seasonal healthy fruits and vegetables. On the weekends you can find me riding shotgun in my husband's truck to pick up some of the freshest produce grown in Southern California. During the off-season, we do sell produce from other parts of the world. It's sort of exciting to sell oranges flown in from Australia or cherries from Chile. I have learned firsthand which produce you should try to buy organic and which ones you really don't have to worry about. You would be surprised at some of the remedial questions customers will ask when they are trying to appear like an expert on the fruit they're buying from thumping the fruit to thinking cherries should be in season all year round in California. (Most clients forget that all fruits and vegetables are seasonal wherever they are growing.) But then again, I didn't know most of these facts either until I married into a wonderful family of farmers. This idyllic fruit stand can be found in the affluent enclave of Rancho Santa Fe, which is a community in the San Diego area. Set against the backdrop of rolling hillsides, Lemon Twist – the name of the business – resonates deep in my heart because of my original roots from being raised on a farm in Southern Missouri. I think that may be one of the reasons I love Lemon Twist so much, besides the obvious – I love my husband.

Over the last few years, I have consciously focused on eating real foods versus processed and packaged food. (Although I will reveal my one exception to that rule.) In my quest to stay healthy, I have discovered some must-haves on my grocery list that factor into the Middle Age Beauty equation. These suggestions also include a couple of tips on what to drink, eat for breakfast, and also find out what I eat when I am craving sweets!

Food and Drink Tips to help manage your waistline

Yams: Did you know that yams are grown in Africa, South America and the Mediterranean? I didn't until I started researching the benefits of why they are just so good for you. I always thought they were grown in America. You might have, too. So it's a good chance that the yam you think you are eating is actually a red sweet potato, which is now called a yam by almost everyone. (Real yams from Africa are not as nutritious as the red sweet potatoes that we eat in America. Since everyone refers to red sweet potatoes as yams, I am referencing the American version.) Did you know that one yam can contain up to 30% of your daily vitamin C needs? Yams are also listed as one of the 'Super Foods', because they are packed full of so many nutrients and vitamins. One medium-sized yam also has up to six grams of fiber. They are also an excellent source of potassium and vitamin B. My favorite perk about the yam is that they are low on the Glycemic Index, which means great news for all of us. (The Glycemic Index is a chart that shows how food can spike our blood sugar. Low on the index is considered best.) As a complex carbohydrate, yams are filling and most of all delicious. So don't wait until Thanksgiving to add these to your list. Add them every week as a source of excellent nutrition, an easy meal to prepare as a side dish, or a stand-alone snack that can give you extra energy to finish out the rest of your day.

Strawberries: Have you ever noticed how eating strawberries just makes you feel happy from just one bite? Maybe it's the bold color of the berry or the fact that we've seen them advertised on our favorite cereals on television commercials. Whatever the actual reason, the world is in love with strawberries. Well, at least Californians are. Did you know California alone as a state produces one billion pounds a year? Wow! Now that's a lot of strawberries. These fat, delicious berries are packed full of antioxidants that aid in eye care, fighting arthritis, gout, and cancer. Eating a large amount of these berries has been proven to reduce the growth of cancerous cells. One tip for those that have a sweet tooth. Try dark chocolate-covered berries for a delicious treat. While tasting remarkably 'sinful', a dark chocolate strawberry registers low on the Glycemic Index and comes in at only 60 calories each!

Greek Yogurt: Go for the Greek Yogurt if you can. My personal favorite is FAGE. From being a probiotic to having live cultures that help our digestive system, yogurt is the perfect in between meal snack, too. Dr. Mike Moreno, the *New York Times* Bestselling author of *The 17 Day Diet* incorporates this yogurt at the beginning of the day and at the end of the day as a way to help promote weight loss naturally. Make sure to steer clear of the yogurts with too much sugar content. Eating yogurt helps strengthen your immune system, too. Some of the other amazing minerals and vitamins found in yogurt include potassium, zinc, vitamin B5 and vitamin B12. So don't skip out on the yogurt section in the grocery store. There are too many important benefits to pass this aisle up.

Drink more water and teas: Cut out all diet colas/energy drinks and switch to Pellegrino/soda water and green or black teas. Most are under the assumption that soda water contains quite a bit of sodium, which makes you retain water. Not true. There is a minimal amount that lends to kicking that afternoon treat you really don't need, while taking in part of your eight glasses of water for the day. Black and green teas are an excellent way to receive your afternoon caffeine jolt, while fighting strokes, too. Yes, that's right. Drinking green and black teas help reduce your risk of ever having a stroke. So make sure you add these to your next grocery list. My main advice here – stop drinking diet sodas! A recent study that just came out linked diet sodas to adding a higher risk of developing the deadly diabetes disease. Many cola companies are now offering much healthier selections today, too. So do cut back on these sugary and aspartame filled drinks. They are truly an enemy when it comes to your health.

Cool Whip: Keep fat-free Cool Whip in your freezer with some frozen berries. If you are like me, it feels pretty fabulous to indulge in a simple sweet tooth fix once on occasion. While I followed my weight loss program, this was my secret trick for having a sugary treat. Of course, don't sit there and eat an obscene amount of blueberries and whipped cream. We're talking an elegant cup at most as your dessert to treat yourself before your evening is over. Okay. This is an obvious, but not a perfect healthy choice here. But if you compare it to eating ½ cup of sugary ice cream, this is an easy way to cut the calories and sugars and enjoy a tasteful treat without overloading your food intake for the day. Cool Whip contains only 25 calories for two tablespoons full! Try real whipped cream, too. (If you don't like whipped cream, try Greek yogurt, with a Truvia packet as a substitute with the berries.) This is more of a 'sweet tooth tip' than a health food tip… the Cool Whip part anyway.

Oatmeal: Eat a small bowl of oatmeal for breakfast. This wasn't actually part of my diet plan. But since I'm a runner, I have found out that this is an excellent source of fiber and 'good carbs' for your body. Add some raisins and some flaxseed, and you have the perfect meal to run 5K in under 28 minutes. While some might tell you that eating steel-cut oats is the only way to go when it comes to eating oatmeal, do not be deterred, instant oatmeal fans. There is only one less grain of fiber per serving. So if you don't have twenty minutes to stir your morning breakfast on the stove, go for the instant packets. I do know there are some low-carb instant oatmeal choices available, too. I personally like the rolled oats by Quaker Oats. They aren't instant, but they are worth that little bit of extra time in the morning because they taste so good. I went through a period where I was obsessing about my oatmeal. One of my girlfriends politely said to me over the phone finally, "Is there anything else going on besides oatmeal?"

I would also like to add lemons, grapefruit, tomatoes and avocadoes to the list of fresh vegetables and fruits that will improve your health by just eating them. From natural fats, cancer fighting fruits to squeezing lemon in your daily dose of water, don't sidestep these must-haves, too. (*Note – if you are trying to lose a significant amount of weight, try adding these after you reach your ideal weight goal.)

Our world is full of choices screaming at us on a daily basis. From Internet to television ads, we are bombarded with daily decisions of what we need to buy and why it will improve our lifestyle. It's up to us though to make the correct choices that can literally add or shave years off our current life span. Do your own research on what foods are great for you. Food is not the enemy. Food is actually good for us. You just have to learn how to be a little more selective though. You might have to have some willpower and learn how to say no… most of the time! Be smart. Think about your health always. Why? Because you deserve it! Yes, that sounds like a soap commercial, but really this time, you do.

Chapter 22

Goodbye Sophistication, Hello Smaller Waistline

Is the movie *Sideways* a movie you strongly identify with because you count yourself a wine connoisseur? Do you enjoy the fact that you know the distinct differences between a Cabernet, a Merlot or a Pinot Noir? Is relaxing to you always connected to unwinding with a glass of Chardonnay or a full-bodied Cab? If you answered yes to any of these questions you may want to read this chapter twice to understand why it's important to choose your health always over the sophisticated looking wine drinker.

A few years back I could have answered all of these questions with a yes, too. I took pride in my wine tasting skills and my happy hour cocktail time with my friends. I drank with glee. This period I am discussing happened in my mid-thirties during that fifteen months of blissful romance with my now husband of four years.

When I began my strict diet that had the restriction of 'no alcohol', I wasn't sure if I would be able to give up my image as the 'sophisticated wine drinker'.

Just like some other women on the planet, I had associated cocktails and full glasses of wine with chic and sexy women living it up in Manhattan. I might not have been walking between skyscrapers every day, but I knew the difference between a full-bodied Cabernet and my favorite Pinot Noir.

After six weeks of not drinking and finding a healthier lifestyle which included a slimmer me, I began to see the difference in my face and also... yes, my wrinkles!

The bloated, tired-looking face that would sometimes look puffy after even just two glasses with my best girlfriends had vanished. The slimmer version of me that resembled my modeling days started reappearing. I noticed my cheekbones again. My flab off my arms had melted with those pounds I had unwittingly gained while living the glamorous, more sophisticated life with my girlfriends.

Some may tell you a glass a day is good for your health? Really? Do you want to count out the average of how many ounces and calories you are adding to your already maxed-out food diet? Do you want to keep making excuses for yourself because drinking wine seems classy and so refined?

You can be that person. I am not. I no longer will ever drink wine again. Full of heavy sugars and loaded with calories, don't fool yourself into thinking this is an excellent source of antioxidants. You can find those antioxidants in dark rich fruits, too. Do you want to keep your vibrancy, your buoyancy, to the color of your cheeks or do you want to have that red fleshed out look of a sophisticated wine drinker?

Really it's your choice. Sophistication or health? Acceptance or that fabulous body plus radiant skin that looks naturally youthful without the help of some chemical peel or fancy face filler. Just like everything in life, your choices make up who you are. My decision to forego wine has had interesting reverberations.

A group of friends of mine that used to meet weekly to share some happy hour wine cocktails finally stopped calling me to join the party. The thing about drinking, if you aren't drinking with the rest of them, there is usually that weird pressure or feeling and those whispers... like, oh is she in AA?

Did she give up alcohol because she had to?

The short answer is: YES. I gave up wine because I found out how absolutely satisfying it was to look younger and feel better! No longer did I wake up with that bloated look. No longer did I see my waistline bulging again because I made a choice that defined something definitive within me.

You could say now that I am a non-drinking wine snob. When

I see others drinking wine, I almost feel sorry for them. I don't think they truly know what they are doing to their overall health.

You may argue that you only drink a couple of glasses with dinner from time to time. What you want to do is start being realistic with yourself and start adding those 'time-to-time' drinks up and do the math on the calorie intake.

Have you weighed yourself lately? Stop drinking for two weeks and weigh in after that. I am rather angered by the pressure still by others to drink socially at parties. I have now come to terms with just always saying 'no thank you' politely without barraging my friends with lectures on why wine could be ruining their skin, their future and adding years of age to their face. No one wants to hear those nitty details at a party. No one wants to hear that the once fun social queen with the fun column in town is now sipping soda water with lime, and no longer is dancing on the tables.

Don't be fooled by the seduction of wine… or your love affair with alcohol. You are no longer 21 or 25 or 30 if you have picked up this book and are looking for cheap aging tips that don't require a visit to a doctor's office, while forking out your hard-earned paycheck. The number one advice I can give any woman looking to shave off years from their face is to just give up all alcoholic beverages.

Take my advice and save a drink or two for *only* special occasions… like a trip with your husband or best friend. Savor those times only once in awhile and watch, many wonderful things will occur.

What wonderful things will happen in my life when I cut out my love for wine?

Besides being an absolute lightweight that can't drink as much, you will soon see that your pocketbook and your checking account will have a larger sum of money in it because you decided to stop partying it up each week with the local number of friends at a place you want to call 'Cheers', except in real life there aren't any paid actors collecting big paychecks and you will definitely be feeling that pounding headache in the morning.

I know. I sound so stodgy. I have become slightly more calm with this realization and understanding of why wine doesn't really amount to sophistication anyway.

Being sophisticated has to do with something within your soul. An air about you, your style, your persona, your being. Don't misconstrue holding a drink in your hand that means you are looking sophisticated, too.

Life isn't a *Sex and the City* rerun. I had to break down my own illusions and aspirations to understand that Carrie Bradshaw and Bridget Jones are just fictional characters that enjoy booze during their emotional bouts; that doesn't mean I have to follow in their fictional shoes.

I had a friend just call me today and ask me, "Are you good? You happy?"
The answer is yes!

I might seem a bit more average without my classy, slender wine glass in hand. But I have found my passion in my health and swearing off unwanted calories that could only complicate my *now* and my *future*.

I know.

That doesn't sound very sexy does it? It doesn't sound sexy to be healthy but then again, there is a new trend going on glamorizing health and it's starting to become the in thing. I just want to see all of these folks that are supposedly buying organic or living the gluten-free diet, if they are still making room for their bottle of Cab or Chardonnay with dinner. When someone preaches to me about gluten when they are busy drinking and cocktailing it up, I begin to wonder what kind of research they have done on wine… or alcohol for that matter.

Here are some statistics you may not want to read

Drinking too much can lead to these fatal health issues. Making small changes to your drinking habits now could not only make you look and feel better, it could also improve your long-term health and well-being. Excessive drinking can lead to these health issues:

Diabetes
Liver disease
Heart disease
Stroke
Immune system
Infertility
Cancer
Memory
High blood pressure
Pancreatitis

There are more than 75,000 deaths a year related to alcohol according to the Centers of Disease Control and Prevention in the US. These statistics are all-important things to remind ourselves before we want to cut loose or unwind too much with the dependency of looking classy.

Remember just like choosing you before you choose your food, the same goes for what you are drinking. Don't be seduced by the advertisements, the taste or the need to fit in. The famous poet Rumi who is idolized for his poetry also said, "Either give me more wine or leave me alone."

Unfortunately, Rumi didn't age well according to those few images we do have left of him from the time during the 12th century, and I am sure back then wrinkles were thought of as badges of courage with each passing year.

You might love his poetry, but don't follow that quote. Take my advice and say goodbye to wine or looking sexy with that slim stem wine glass filled with fermented grapes. Learn to love yourself more.

If you must know my one secret drink that I will allow myself for that special trip with my husband it's – Tequila! Yes, that's right. Sip it, don't shoot it. Try a blanco tequila and make sure it's a decent brand. Tequila does not spike your blood sugar like other wines and alcoholic beverages because it is made from an agave plant. You can look this one up, too. It's an excellent tip for anyone that suffers from blood sugar disorders.

So do picture me once a year in Mexico sipping my delicious tequila wearing a bikini because I was smart enough to say no to that one popular cocktail – a glass of wine. Since I rarely drink now, only on 'special occasions' is so much better for my health.

Okay. So you can't quit wine – then just cut back. Drink less.

At least start counting your glasses. All I can tell you is when I cut this from my diet, my skin, my health and my overall appearance improved so much. I feel like I look much better than I did in my thirties because I was drinking wine back then.

After all, you only have one body, one face, one life and one you. I managed to make the change... can you? Just remember if you are drinking one glass of wine a day, with an average of 100 calories per glass, you are adding 36,500 EXTRA calories a year to your body in one year. So make a point to cut back, slim down and stop being so darn sophisticated.

Chapter 23

The One Shot You Need: Vitamin B Shots

Are you ready to find out which needle you can use for what shot to combat anti-aging? This is the one needle that you should allow yourself one weekly dose of... a vitamin B shot! In 2009, when I went on a regimented diet program that helped me radically change my body, a weekly vitamin B shot was just one of the weekly must-haves on this diet program. Five years later I am still making time for this one important needle to help me feel younger, healthier and more alert every day. While many women in Southern California are making appointments for needles in their forehead and other areas on their face, I am taking my shot at the top of my right hip. Yes, that's right. It's quick. It's painless. And best of all, you feel an immediate boost that enhances not only the rest of your day, also your entire week.

So do me a favor: Choose your needles carefully. Do think before you subject yourself to unneeded fillers that have been reported to travel to other areas in your body, while diminishing your abilities to empathize with your friend or next-door neighbor. Just say no to Botox and say yes to vitamin B shots. The best news is this shot also falls right at the $20.00 price. What's more important than your health? Well, maybe nourishing your soul from the inside out first, but your health is interconnected and should always be at the top of your list.

Why Vitamin B Shots? Should I consult my doctor?

Yes, please know that I am a woman just like you. These suggestions in my book are tips that have worked for me, and I have had positive results. In order to receive a vitamin B shot, you must actually consult with a doctor first. I did. So, you should, too. As a woman in her forties, I have learned some important factors that have helped improve my energy, change my mood and improve my health. Vitamin B shot is at the top of my list for helping me stay healthier and most of all improve my overall sense of well-being.

Vitamin B12 is an energy vitamin. When you receive a shot, you immediately receive a boost of energy to your system. Fighting fatigue and boosting your metabolism are just two effects of this one must-have shot that you need to pencil in onto your calendar. This one five-minute moment of my week just happens to be one of my 'joys' I make time for because I am making time for myself and health. In some areas in California some of the medical spas and homeopathic clinics actually call these shots 'the skinny shot', because the vitamin B shot does help speed up our metabolism. Did you know our metabolism actually begins to slow down at the age of 25?

Wow! Why didn't someone tell me then? You can actually lose up to 20–40% of your metabolic power during your life span. So, this is one important factor to consider especially for men and women over forty, to add vitamin B shots to their to-do lists! How many do I average in a month? I average about three shots a month. This has radically helped me in other ways besides boosting my metabolism. My energy and my mood, plus my overall health have been an average A grade, which is high for me.

A few years ago, I had the opportunity of profiling Dr. Kim Kelly, an expert in homeopathic medicine in Southern California. I have frequented his clinic on numerous occasions over the last few years for my vitamin B shot. As a licensed Naturopathic Doctor in the state of California, he has been an advocate and promoter of the effectiveness of alternative therapies toward health.

Here is my interview with Dr. Kim Kelly:

Dr. Kelly, what would you say the number one benefit is for women and men over forty to start taking vitamin B shots?

What do your patients tell you are their most immediate benefits they receive?

Dr. Kelly: The number one benefit is the improvement in their energy – this is due to the fact that the B-vitamins are essential to the conversion of food energy (into ATP), which is the form of energy your cells use. As we age, the amount of vitamins and minerals we absorb decreases. This is further compounded if people have gut issues. By getting a vitamin B shot, this helps to ensure adequate levels in the body. Taking B-vitamins orally is beneficial, but research has shown that getting B-vitamin injections have shown a significant improvement in well-being and health compared to those taking it orally.

Do you see a direct correlation between weight loss and the vitamin B shot?

Dr. Kelly: This varies for each person. The B-vitamins are necessary for metabolism of fats, carbohydrates and proteins. Getting the vitamin B shots do help to increase metabolism. However, getting B-vitamin shots alone is not the way to lose weight. If combined with right diet, exercise and proper lifestyle, you have a good program for success in losing weight. Also, one should have their hormones checked too, as another reason might be low thyroid function.

What are some of the other positive perks of adding vitamin B shots to a person's health regimen?

Dr. Kelly: Because the B-vitamins help with so many functions in the body, there are many benefits besides weight loss and energy. B-vitamins are water-soluble vitamins that dissolve easily in water and are transported throughout your body in your bloodstream. The B-vitamins all work together to support our immune system, promote cell growth and division, skin and muscle health maintenance and improve nerve function. For example, some people report much better sleep after getting the B12-cocktail shot. Other people have better ability to focus after getting a B12-cocktail shot. The B12 (methylcobalamin) is needed to help in detoxing the pathway in the liver.

I find when I am receiving my regular vitamin B shots that my mood is more cheerful and optimistic. Do vitamin B shots also help with boosting your mood and overall health?

Dr. Kelly: The vitamin B shots help with mood as it helps with serotonin levels. Serotonin is the 'happy' neurotransmitter and B6 is needed to help make this. Also, plenty of research has shown people with depression often have low B12 levels. The brain uses B1 (thiamin) to help convert glucose, or blood sugar, into fuel, and without it the brain rapidly runs out of energy. This can lead to fatigue, depression, irritability and anxiety. Deficiencies of the B-vitamins can also cause memory problems, loss of appetite, insomnia, and gastrointestinal disorders.

What encouraging words would you say to someone that is uncertain of trying a vitamin B shot for the first time? Are there any downsides to a vitamin B shot?

Dr. Kelly: I use a small gauge needle so people will basically just feel a tiny pinch when I give them a B shot. It is more the anticipation of the shot that makes it feel painful, than the shot itself. After the B shot, they are surprised how easy it was. There are some people who may get a small rash or feel an itch at the site of the B12 shot but it resolves after a day or two.

What are the advantages of taking a shot versus taking supplements? Do you think that individuals over forty benefit significantly from a vitamin B shot?

Dr. Kelly: When taking B-vitamins orally, many factors can affect the absorption. People lacking intrinsic factors have a very difficult time absorbing B12 if taken orally. People under stress often do not have efficient absorption of their nutrients. As we age, especially after age 50, the amount of vitamins we absorb is going to be less than when we were in our 20s and 30s. When getting a vitamin B shot, one has 100% absorption, and for people who are deficient, they will feel a dramatic boost in their energy and well-being.

I have found adding these shots once weekly to my schedule have been overall beneficial to improving my health, my weight and most of all my sense of well-being. What is your recommendation on how many a month you would suggest a patient to try, and why?

Dr. Kelly: The typical protocol for vitamin B shots is once a week for four weeks as the loading dose and then monthly as maintenance dose. However, people most often come once a month for the vitamin B shot as it is easier on their schedule. For those who do come once a week, they notice how it helps maintain their energy, their moods and their overall well-being. For patients wanting that extra boost to help lose weight, I add in what's called MIC with the B-vitamins. The MIC is called the 'fat burner' and stands for: Methionine (an amino acid), Inositol (a co-factor) and Choline (a co-factor). When getting the MIC with the B-vitamin shot, it is helpful to get this every week.

What's wonderful about this shot is you actually feel an immediate boost. With society so driven for that instant fix, this is definitely one that should attract many. And the best news is it's something your body needs. Especially as we grow older and hit our Middle Age Beauty period.

So remember the next time you consider taking a needle to the forehead… *don't!* Get a vitamin B shot instead. After all, it's the one shot that receives my stamp of approval for your health and your beauty.

Key factors to take with you from this chapter:

The one needle that's good for you – a Vitamin B shot.

Vitamin B shots help boost your mood and your immune system.

Vitamin B shots also boost your metabolism.

Chapter 24

Why 15 Minutes or Less Can Help You Work Out More

15 minutes or less is one of the most recognizable catch phrases today, from commercials to smart phones giving updates for our reminders. You know the one with the cute green gecko lizard with the English accent? This commercial actually came about because of an actors' strike in Hollywood in 1999. Sometimes brilliance is born out of a circumstance that forces you to find a new creative route. This one slogan is easily recognized and sticks in your mind. From the visual of the green lizard to the repetitive number 15, you don't forget it. Fifteen minutes doesn't sound like much time and your mind accepts it as a doable number that can fit into your schedule. From 15-minute breaks, at the office, to 15 minute daily notification buzz, this number makes sense to our schedule.

The year I turned forty also happened to be the year I hit runner's burnout. I had been into running off and on at different periods of my life. From subscribing to *Runner's World* magazine to reading running books, this was the one exercise my mind and body craved. But just like anything you repetitively do too much of, there is a significant chance you will need to take a break.

Instead of running my short runs, I decided to walk. In the mornings after dropping my son off at school, trust me the last thing I wanted to do was even walk because I was feeling the burnout. That's when I realized the value of this slogan. This 15 minutes or less commercial could be applied to my workouts. I found if I suggested to myself the workout will only last this short amount of time, I would usually still get in a workout before the day started. The great news is I honestly would always walk about 30 minutes in the morning. And even then sneak in some sprints to mix it up a bit. After one solid year of doing minor workouts compared to long endurance runs, I was completely surprised that I was still in decent shape by the time my next birthday appeared on the calendar. Who knew? In the beginning of the Millennium in 2002, *Time Magazine* published an article by Christine Gorman, "Walk, Don't Run".

When did the walking craze hit? Well there are reports of it actually making strides in 1979, pre-dating the *Let's Get Physical* phase with Olivia Newton John's aerobic tights by three years. Just like any exercise trend, they come and go... and are rediscovered.

After doing some research on why walking was just as marvelous as running as far as my physique goes, I found out that I was still clocking in enough time and energy at a decent pace to still have the desired effects as running. (No offense to any runners. I still love running. I'm just learning to appreciate my surroundings more, while enjoying some cardio in the morning.)

So back to the 15 minutes. Do you have 15 minutes in the morning to improve your life?

I bet you do. I'm sure your mind can figure out a way to organize yourself the night before by having your workout clothes ready to go so you are able to sneak in those 15 minutes or less for who... You!

Here are just some of the benefits you can receive by incorporating walking into your weekly routine:
- Weight control and weight loss.
- Fights heart disease. The heart is considered a muscle and needs to be exercised much like our body does. So forget about weight control, think about the importance of keeping your heart healthy... especially since that is the number one killer among men and women.

- Walking helps lower our blood pressure.
- Can keep diabetes at bay. Consistent exercise of at least 15 minutes in the morning and in the evening (if you need to break up the time) can actually help prevent your chances of developing this deadly disease, which has become an epidemic in America. According to the American Diabetes Association if current trends continue in America, one in every three Americans will develop diabetes by the year 2050. That's a staggering statistic that you don't want to become a part of... ever!
- Walking is also known to help improve your mood and fight depression.

This may seem like a low amount of exercise that will not be enough to keep you in shape. Believe it or not, this is better than doing nothing.

Most of tend to think of working out as an hour experience at the gym. And sometimes 60 minutes just seems like too much time for us to squeeze into our day. So remember, the ultimate goal is to work out longer, however to 'trick' your mind into thinking it's only going to be 15 minutes.

Applying the 15-minute theory to your workout can also help you incorporate other exercises you can do in the comfort of your own home. If you don't have time or the little extra cash for the gym, no problem. Dial up your smart phone. Yes, that's right. At your fingertips is a personal trainer with several apps that you can download for free to your phone which can help you get in shape without spending extra money on a personal trainer. But do make sure you stick to your schedule.

This is how I break my workout week down so it's not the same repetitive action every day. I choose from these options so I can at least work out three to four times a week.

- Schedule three to four morning walks a week. If you have

a dog, make sure you give your pet their exercise, too. They need it just as much as you do!

- Do a series of sit-ups and push-ups with your weekly free apps on your smart phone. These training programs are easy to follow and allow mini-breaks between your sets… and even have whistle blowing to notify you when to start next.

- Squats – I just discovered this amazing exercise that you can do anywhere, anytime even in most of your normal dress clothes… excluding those tight miniskirts or the days you are wearing your ultra skinny jeans. Trust me, you might split those if you do your squats in them. How do I know, because I have had this happen to me.

- Work out at the gym. I just recently joined a gym again so I can incorporate spinning and weight training at least two to three times a week as a break. I am only spending $35.00 a month toward improving my health, excitement and choices in my workout routine. One of the major benefits of working out at a gym is being surrounded by others that are motivated to stay fit. One of my top rock star spin instructors – Kris – is my inspiration. Her body is an 11 and I am always amazed at her dedication to working out, her mental attitude and her contagious enthusiasm that spreads to all of us in her class. Working out in a gym is also a mini-getaway from your family. Remember it's important to take time for yourself so you have enough energy to give your best performance in other areas in your life.

- Find a walking partner.

- Rescue a dog. Besides being good for the soul, owning a dog can do wonders for your health. Walking a dog is a must as a pet owner. And if you need extra motivation to leap off the couch into your tennis shoes, trust me, a dog will definitely help you do it. Their little pleading by the door next to their leash will be something you can't pass up.

- Buy five-pound weights and keep them in your bedroom. One true sign of age – especially for women – can be flabby, saggy arms. Listen, fellow women friends, do not let this happen to you! Keep your arms nice and toned by doing a few sets of twenty in the morning before the day starts, and in the evening before you go to bed. Nothing looks sexier on a woman than when she can walk out of the house in a Sigourney Weaver-looking T-shirt (think the *Alien* series here), complemented by a pair of worn-in Levi's. The investment is also under $20.00 for your health. (We lose body muscle mass as we grow older.)

- Stretch. Don't forget to stay limber. Stretching is important for our body and our health. Yes, yoga can be inserted here, too. I have incorporated some simple yoga moves that I can easily do after my sit-ups, which help me stay limber and flexible. You don't want to become stiff and brittle with age. So remember to stretch.

Okay so maybe it's a bit odd a green lizard with an English accent helped reinvent my workout routine into a more appealing and diversified one by simply applying that 15 minutes or less theory. Remember the next time you think you don't have enough time to exercise, play that small trick on your mind to see if it works for you. The trick is to just get up and move! Get creative and don't become a boring couch potato because you think it's okay since you are now over 45 and your metabolism has slowed down. Now is the time more than ever to just… *walk!*

Chapter 25

Omega 3 and Fish Oil Pills

Okay. Yes, I am guilty. I have been one of those individuals that have put on unwanted weight, while enjoying the good life. In my younger years I could literally eat a cheeseburger for dinner and never think twice about the ramifications of weight gain from calorie intake or from saturated fats. I haphazardly made it through most of my twenties and early thirties with no thought whatsoever worrying about the number on a scale beneath my feet. I even lost all of my baby weight easily because I was an active runner that lived and breathed the excitement of shaving off a minute of a fast-paced mile.

Well, that was all before I hit 35.

Yes, that little number does seem to be a big one in the cycle, especially for women. From having our eggs downgraded by quality and experiencing a ghostly ticking clock in our body telling us to produce a baby, this one particular number is easy to recognize as a milestone birthday. Whether we like it or not, as a woman or man we need to make healthier lifestyle choices if we want to live a more fulfilling life. Patricia Bragg wrote in her book *Apple Cider Vinegar: Miracle Health System* that you are either on the road to sickness and disease, or on the road to health.

Which road are you on? I wish I could say I have been on this road from the beginning of my adulthood, but at least I discovered it by applying action to the error of my ways.

So you can imagine the humiliation I felt when I did succumb to the weight loss program monitored by a doctor. Luckily for me, I was smart enough to acknowledge that I needed to lose weight, and did not hide behind my ignorance and avoid a scale. I actually refused to get on the scale on my first visit for this program. It took me two months to swallow my pride and my ego to see that maybe there was something I needed to learn about my diet now that I did not know on my own.

So seeking a nutritionist and doctor's help was one of the smartest lifestyle choices I ever made. I discovered how to eat healthy without doing some extreme yo-yo diet. I learned that what I place in my mouth just doesn't miraculously burn away at the gym if I am eating more calories than I am taking in... so if you need some redirection, seek help! If this sounds pricey, do some research online and compare your current lifestyle to the recommendations you find. Do you need to make some changes now, too?

It's never easy admitting we may need help with something. But once you do, you will also benefit from the boost in your self-esteem for knowing your mind, body and soul are worth making your number one priority. So if you are smoking... quit! If you are drinking too much... stop. If you are a binge eater, find help. If you don't feel good about the way you look, don't worry. Baby steps will lead you to the way of the ultimate goal you may have in mind.

Making a strenuous effort to live a healthier lifestyle can actually be a positive and fun experience.

What is the most rewarding though is feeling and looking great every day. Which brings me to one of my last important, easy tips that can help improve your health and well-being. What if you knew that taking a couple of Omega 3/fish oil pills could help improve the positivity of the outcome of your day? Does that sound farfetched to you? Well, if you happen to be over the age of forty or in the midst of your middle-aged years this is a chapter you should definitely not skip over. Many times we think that we can receive most of our nutrients from our food. However, in a realistic, chaotic world, there's a good chance you are not eating salmon every day of the week to obtain this important fatty acid and fish oil.

I know. This is not that exciting. Fish oil and Omega 3 pills. *What is exciting is* to discover and find out the importance of just how this supplement is an important one to add to your list today.

I discovered the importance of Omega 3/fish oil pills when I was approached by a doctor in Rancho Santa Fe to be monitored on his diet and nutrition plan. As I have already written in an earlier chapter, this program helped introduce me to living a healthier lifestyle.

The odds are you may already be taking Omega 3s every day because you know that this helps reduce your cholesterol levels. But did you also know that this supplement helps improve your overall health, fights depression and improves your energy levels, while curbing your appetite?

I didn't.

Before I uncover your next tip, let's break down what the key important health tips are in the Health section:

- Melatonin
- Bragg's Apple Cider Vinegar
- Avoid drinking wine and alcohol in general
- Follow a healthy lifestyle plan
- Discard colas and diet colas for flavored waters and teas
- Choose your food wisely
- Work out at least 15 minutes three to five times a week
- Weigh in with yourself. Jump on a scale and find out what you weigh
- Take Omega 3/Fish Oil pills

One of the most exciting aspects of writing this book has been the opportunity to interview experts in the field of health and psychology. I found my sources by applying some of my important health decisions that have dramatically improved my health.

Lauren Antonucci is the owner of Nutrition Energy in New York City. She is well respected as a nationally acclaimed nutritionist. Her impressive athletic background includes thirteen marathons, numerous triathlons and Ironman USA – three times. I discovered Lauren by reading one of my favorite magazines, *Runner's World*. She has been featured for her writing and as a nutritional expert in the *New York Times*, *Diabetes Self-Management*, plus many more. I had the privilege of interviewing Lauren regarding three important health questions that women over forty need to know. On a side note, what I find most inspiring about Lauren is she is also a mother of three children, while being a bona fide rock star in the fitness and nutritional world to many.

Here is my interview with Lauren Antonucci:

What is a common mistake women make when they are dieting? Specifically geared to women forty and older?

Lauren Antonucci: Most women during their midlife period are not getting enough Omega 3 fats, and cut out good fats from their diet, which is a mistake. Women need to invest calories in the good fats because they help boost your energy and your mood, which is essential to your daily activities. Your energy and mood contribute to your overall well-being.

- Walnuts
- Omega 3s
- Two tablespoons full of fish oils

These are good examples of how to add healthy fat into your daily diet.

As a nutritionist and health expert you counsel many clients about changing or adding to daily food intake? In what other areas can women improve their diet?

Lauren Antonucci: Women do not eat enough fiber in their diet. This helps contribute to a healthier digestive system. Spread your fiber out during the daytime. Do not eat it all at once. Do eat your fiber in natural foods like oranges, fruits and legumes. These are the best natural sources for eating fiber.

Do you think eating healthy can help you contribute to staying naturally young?

Lauren Antonucci: Yes. Anti-aging foods are the darkest you can get your hands on: dark greens, reds, purples… these are all considered anti-aging – while loaded with antioxidants. So incorporate these into your daily consumption of food.

After my interview with Lauren, I called all of my girlfriends and urged them to start eating the good fats. Don't cut them out. Take those Omega 3/fish oil pills each day just in case you are not eating enough natural fats on your own. Our energy and our mood affect our actions, our communication and how we interact with others. So don't glaze over little measures like eating good fats. Don't ignore healthy steps that are easy to incorporate into your diet. Don't ignore your health. Like in the classic movie, *The Princess Bride*, with many memorable lines, one applies perfectly here: "If you haven't got your health, then you haven't got anything." Thank you to all of the experts in this important section of *Middle Age Beauty* for sharing your expert advice. You may be helping someone discover that with the right choices and actions, the second half of their lifetime can indeed be their best!

Part Three – Your Beauty

There's nothing tragic about being fifty. Not *unless* you're *trying to be twenty-five.*
~ *Sunset Boulevard*, Billy Wilder, Charles Brackett and DM Marshman, Jr.

Chapter 26

Your Beauty

What is beauty? The definition of beauty according to the Oxford dictionary says:

The combination of qualities such as shape and color or form that pleases the aesthetic senses, especially the sight.

Some might say that cliché saying 'beauty is only skin deep'.

Beauty resonates deep from within first, while our exterior also illuminates our soul.

Our body is to be treasured and to be treated with respect and love. I've heard all sorts of theories now regarding women over forty and how they should act and behave. I have had certain acquaintances say to me in brief discussion, "What is the point? Can't we just admit we are older and throw in the towel?" There is nothing to admit. There is nothing to counter. There is only you. How you take care of yourself from the inside and out is ultimately your choice.

If you feel like you don't care enough about your personal looks and this is not a goal for you because you have made thousands of excuses, like you are now living during your midlife chapter – *now* is the time to reassess your thinking and replace your thoughts with more magical and light thoughts. Don't you want to be the *hero of your own story*, like Mary McCarthy suggests? I do!

You can *'take time to make time'* for your daily beauty habits. Beauty isn't just about your skin care or your weight size. Beauty is a personal decision to make yourself a priority. Why? When you look in the mirror you can say, "Wow that's me? I like her. I'm taking care of her and I feel better about myself because I am taking time to nourish my soul, health and beauty each day." I am no longer placing my needs on an excuse list. I am making myself a top priority.

I remember when I was nineteen years old and I moved to San Francisco for a few months at the early stages of my modeling career. Imagine a semi-tall gangly dirty dishwater blonde wearing stonewashed jeans, high top tennis shoes and bright neon pink lipstick. When I checked in with my agent, Kim, inside this cool trendy loft just down from where the trolleys operate in the center of the town, I was a bit shell-shocked with the first words out of her mouth to me:

"Oh, honey, we have to do something about the way you look. You can't be going around town like that. And, you must get some eyebrows immediately!"

"I have eyebrows, right?" I shyly retorted.

"No, you don't. You can't see them. They are blonde. Your face looks like a white plate."

Oh.

To this day, I tell those I know that my face looks like a white plate without my brows darkened with either eyebrow pencil or color. Being a real blonde does have its drawbacks I guess. (Although, yes, I am guilty of highlighting it to a few shades lighter since I'm a Marilyn Monroe fan!) I also found out some basics on how to dress at that time, appropriately as a model, and let's just say the stonewashed jeans and high tops were never seen in public again. I will also let you know that this time period was during the height of Billy Idol, when Patrick Swayze was the most famous poster for teenagers and a rock group named U2 still hadn't found what they were looking for...

I look back on those days... I am grateful I had someone being blunt and honest with me. I will admit to you that I did go back to the model's flat and cry a few silent tears of embarrassment.

Twenty years later the world has changed so much. It's much

easier for a young girl from a farm in the Midwest to stay current on style than it was back then due to the technology explosion. Don't worry, I am not going to be telling you how to dress or what trends are in. However, I will tell you that there are simple classic themes that never change. We will discuss later on that one. This will be your own personal choice if you accept my advice or if you think it's not your cup of tea.

Your outward appearance is a signal to others on what you feel about yourself. So if your shoestring is untied or your jeans have that 'hole effect' you may be conveying that you are lackadaisical and uninspiring. So make sure how you dress is really the statement you want to promote about yourself. If you are thinking here that you are just too lazy to care, you definitely need to read this section. Living in a pair of 'mom sweats' because you are too busy may be affecting your life and your mood more than you think. This is truly an important part of the beauty trinity for you to read and to go over honestly with yourself. I am a self-promoter. I believe in promoting those I love, too.

Beauty is linked to our health and soul. Our outward appearance is our first impression to others whether we like it or not. What do how you dress and your skin say about yourself? Do you know? If you don't, I want you to spend time finding out and analyzing your style and your daily attitude toward beauty. The naysayers and those that would want you to believe you are shallow for caring about your outward appearance aren't telling you the fundamental truths of how society works and why this should be on your number one agenda. Whether you like it or not, your personal appearance matters. What you wear can define how others perceive you.

In this section I will be sharing with you simple tips and dispelling certain myths that women face with age.

I will go over some simple beauty suggestions and products

that will help rejuvenate your outward appearance with simple tricks that can save you money and keep your skin looking younger longer... *the natural way.* These products do not involve hazardous injections of any kind. You might even be surprised when you find out my number one skin secret that I have followed religiously now for fifteen years. I will suggest some simple routine habits that can affect you from the inside out. These activities are easy to incorporate into your week. It only requires making some time for the most important person in your life – *you!* I will discuss your appearance, what it means and why what you wear should not be based on fashion trends or trying to look more mature with age. Learn why the great outdoors can add to your radiant glow. Estée Lauder once said:

Beauty is an attitude. There is no secret... There are no ugly women. Only women who don't care or don't believe they're attractive.

Are you ready to check in with your beautiful self? After all, there is only one beautiful *you.*

Chapter 27

Develop Your Persona

Are you feeling confident and secure about yourself? If you aren't, chances are the rest of the world knows it, too. There could be worse things in life. However, since your best friend should be *you* first, are you making sure you are giving *her* the best you can each day?

 During my mid-twenties I faced one of those heart-wrenching scary times when the world stops making sense, life fell flat and my attitude lacked that confidence and upbeat attitude I always had just naturally. Hollywood has a way of unraveling any sane person into a person feeling frazzled. From thousands of acting classes, to self-help bookstores to finding your bliss, that town has every token for you to find and which then offers a quick solution. *Except for me none of them worked…*

Maybe I was too much of that 'good girl' from the Midwest that still believed in deeper things than finding a new tattoo parlor or hot yoga. Since my arrival to the acting scene had been more from my modeling side, I found myself standing at a crossroads at 27 with no backbone, no bookings and absolute sheer lack of attitude. I had relinquished them somewhere between my hundreds of auditions requiring me to scream, "Pick me! I'm the right girl for the part!"

After seven years of schlepping and running around Hollywood with my beeper and a Thomas Guide, I felt exhausted from exerting so much exterior confidence to the world. What I found out when my foundation of confidence collapsed underneath me was that I had some serious work to do regarding finding why and how this had happened to me. Well my *persona* had turned out to be a young girl maybe not tough enough for the acting business. I found this out only as I was actually *exiting* the city. Yes, that's right. Sometimes we learn crucial information when it's too late. But it's still good to find out the truth.

When I turned 27, I moved to San Diego with my first husband. After delving into why there was something missing for me under the bright lights of the big city, I remembered that I had only originally stepped foot onto the stage because that was what my modeling agents had suggested. "You have a commercial face, you should also go into acting." Okay! Why not, I remember thinking?

Well seven years later my experience had me on a soul-searching mission to figure out my 'right path'. So I went on my own personal deeper search within myself and found what I truly wanted had more to do with family and writing than booking acting jobs for a GM car commercial. When I realized my persona was more of what my soul resembled and less of what I should have been portraying to book more acting jobs, instead of being upset with myself for not showing a tougher exterior, I found myself feeling oddly proud that I never altered who I innately was just to climb the ladder of success.

Persona. What does that mean? Do you know? Persona is someone's outward character perceived by others. This means basically: How others view you in their eyes. So back to my discovery of my persona before moving from Los Angeles.

Upon leaving Hollywood to move to the San Diego area, I had a frank conversation with my manager at the Hamburger Hamlet on Wilshire in Beverly Hills. We ordered fat burgers and thinly-cut fries. While waiting for our burgers to arrive with the side of fries, I nervously sat across from the woman I admired, revered and respected more than anyone. I hated the fact that I was disappointing her because I was moving to San Diego. I dreaded our conversation as much as the high lofty ceilings in this trendy upscale burger hangout. (Bad acoustics and always super loud.) Finally she began talking loudly over the noise as we began our conversation.

"Well, Machel, if I could have heard any other words than what a nice girl you were that would been so much better than always hearing the word… *nice.*"

"What words were you hoping for?" I was totally stumped. (Imagine me still just in my mid-twenties too green to even get this conversation!)

"Interesting maybe… edgy… I would have even gone for weird. Anything but nice. That's what the casting agents would always say to me. Machel is so nice… you were too nice for Hollywood, Machel."

Well, this made sense. My ears perked up. I smelled the delicious aroma of the burgers wafting from the back of the kitchen. I understood for the first time that my agent and I had different ideas of what was important and valuable in this life. Bargaining away part of who I was to land more face commercials or print ads just had never been something I had ever considered. A warm smile met her blank stare. I was still being too nice I think… but I was beginning to have one of those moments where you feel like the cameras *should be* rolling. I had finally arrived for myself and felt suddenly alert and poised. I suddenly wished Francis Ford Coppola could have been there for my *Godfather* moment.

I finally replied: "I'm glad I'm a nice girl and if that's not what Hollywood wants, then that's not for me because I'm never changing. I like who I am."

"That's nice, Machel, it doesn't matter because you are moving anyway."

"Yes, that's right. I'm moving," I said smiling from cheek to cheek.

There we were. Two women that had been intertwined with the same dream only to be torn apart by one little word that means absolutely everything: *Persona.*

My persona was being a nice girl. According to her, it was a good thing I was moving to San Diego with my then husband and pregnant with my soon-to-be son. She literally looked at me almost like the first moment she had met me five years before – like I was still green and naïve without learning the fundamental skills to adapt and change in Hollywood.

I wanted to rightly remind her I had still booked over twenty commercials, booked guest starring roles and had my own lead in an independent movie. Not to mention the three-act play I had written got picked up by the HBO Workspace theatre to be showcased… I guess being nice sometimes booked the roles, too. Parting ways with those we love is never easy. And even though I hadn't agreed with her on this one point, I count myself lucky to have had this amazing woman in my life as my manager. She was truly one of the rare breeds of women that was a trailblazer for other women, too. She also encouraged my writing. I was so lucky to spend time with her under the bright, hot lights of Los Angeles.

Overall she was right, though. I never ran around claiming stardom. I ran around hoping the casting directors would like me. I wanted to be nice, shake hands and get to know them. My manager had made a precise judgment about this 'nice girl bit'. She was quite accurate and astute when it came to her judgment.

That seems to be my overall persona I present to the world.

NICE

This can be a blessing and a curse. My experience in Los Angeles molded my character in unexpected ways. Instead of becoming jaded and bitter, I managed to hold on to the real me, while exhausting all efforts on the outward front.

To this day I have this little thing where some consider me too nice and I think that that's okay. I tend to want to scatter sunshine and less of my boldness. I tend to shine in smaller ways than big bold strokes of genius. (Although my closest friends know I can be quite a tough cookie when it comes down to it.)

So let's uncover your Persona

Do you have any idea how others see you? Are there any recurring words that you hear repeated to describe your personality? Can you identify them? If you can't sum up what others think or feel about how you are, then you need to try to do this for yourself.

The overall point on the persona is just this: Be Yourself. Don't change. Share your light. Your energy. Your laughter. Your attitude and demeanor influence your natural beauty. How you carry yourself and speak to others is part of your journey. Are you representing the person you want to be?

If you are confident enough to share the true you on the inside you can simplify your lifestyle by not having to change gears. Define what you want to be from the outside in to others. That is one gift we always have at our fingertips. So what, I come off too nice and that doesn't always gain the right sort of respect. I like who I am and would prefer to be more pleasant than right when it comes to interacting with others. This may not be you. If your soul is more bold, own it baby! Go for the gold. Go for what's inside.

Now take time and write down three words to define who you are. Here are my words that describe me as an example:

Energetic

Optimistic

Light-hearted

Nice

Opinionated

Gentle

Dreamer

Fierce when necessary

Honing in on your persona and how you present yourself to the public is something you can cultivate just like your appearance.

My advice is dare to be your dynamic *you*.

Don't spend time developing a 'fake persona' to share with others. Have the courage to stand alone, to be 'the nice guy' if that's who you are and dare to be you. Your beautiful self is worth sharing. If you can be bold enough to be *original*, then you are going to lock in one key ingredient to your own natural beauty: just being yourself. After all, your persona is the only one that you've got! Unless you are Sybil – then you will need a psychotherapist for that.

Chapter 28

My Secret Weapon in Fighting Wrinkles

Okay, let's be frank. If you can, take my advice and stay natural. I know many women out there have had Botox at a minimal amount. They don't look like they've had some strange face plant with mounds for cheeks and lips that curl up at an odd angle. You know, those lips where you find yourself staring at the corner of their mouth instead of their eyes? Their lips are so wide and puffed up, you wonder if it's actually painful to smile. Take my advice and don't go for that look. You automatically detract from your natural beauty. Be a puritan if you can. Opt for other options that aren't defined by the word 'filler'. If you think I'm one of those women that might be afraid of needles, you are mistaken. I like acupuncture. I like my vitamin B shots. I don't mind a needle. What's inside though, now that's another story.

Watch out for those medical spas that promise you youth by a needle. Instead, if you must, visit one and do a noninvasive treatment like a facial that can be rejuvenating to your skin. Now it's time to get down to the real topic at hand… like what in the world was that 99 cent product in my purse that works even better than Botox?

In the next chapters, I will outline the aging issue we deal with and what products I use to help minimize wrinkles, dark spots and how to keep sun damage to a minimum.

Be ready to be shocked, horrified and have access to your running shoes or a good pair of flip flops because the best news is it's at every grocery store in most countries around the world.

My Top Secret Weapon to combat wrinkles, crow's feet, lip lines and the dreaded squished forehead: Vaseline *with Vitamin E.*

Your Cost: $1.00 to $5.50 depending on the size of the Vaseline container.

Why it works: This is not rocket science really. What Vaseline is made out of is a thick substance that won't even penetrate your skin. It stays on the surface and acts as a shield against the free radicals in the environment.

Most of us add wrinkles to our face every night as we sleep. If you can't sleep perfectly in the bed on your back, then your skin is squishing up against the pillow, while you are sleeping. Now I have one simple question for you. How old are you? How many nights are there in a year and multiply that against your age. What does that equal? A natural progression of wrinkles over time all because of your sleeping position.

Dry skin also adds and increases the visibility of wrinkles. Facial expressions which I discussed in the 'Meditation versus Botox' section are also natural wrinkle producers. So grab that mirror and start monitoring your expressions. Keep your smile light and don't furrow your brow. When you are driving, don't brood over issues that might be stressing you out.

Relax, try to be less stressed and now let's get back to Vaseline.

How to Use – I use Vaseline with vitamin E every night. I apply it to my crow's feet area, above my mouth and my forehead after I use my moisturizer. Do I use a little? No. I use a lot. I do this at the very end of the night right before I go to bed. I wouldn't suggest using it as just your only moisturizer all over your face. However, once a week I do apply Vaseline like I would my moisturizer in heavy amounts from the top of my forehead (I pin my hair back with bobby pins on this night) to the base of my neck. I will tell you that the next morning your face absolutely glows and radiates from this one night intervention from a product that only costs you one dollar. Yes. It's Vaseline.

I know. Your friends and your medical spa clinic will laugh in your face if you tell them your trick. So my advice is carry one small tube in your purse at all times hidden inside the small zipper pouch so it doesn't fall out at your next lady luncheon.

Apply in the morning, too: After washing your face in the morning and applying your light sunscreen protectant, just add a little Vaseline in your most vulnerable wrinkle spots, then cover with your makeup. If I can remember I apply this once or twice during the day.

How I made the discovery:

In 2005, I happened to be a skin care consultant for a few months for a very natural skin care line. I used to host fabulous little parties in my condo with other housewives looking for a reprieve from the almighty wrinkle. My neighbors were willing to try and buy this product that 'worked on a cellular level' that penetrated the skin.

I must tell you at this period in my life I was sort of becoming freaked out by the new creases forming around my eyes like everyone feels, so I thought this whole new skin care journey would be fun, great girl time, while fighting wrinkles.

During this period I just happened to catch an *Oprah Winfrey* episode on television. I say 'catch' because I was literally flipping through the channels and stopped when I read "Secrets to the Fountain of Youth". Where do I sign up for that, I thought.

This particular episode highlighted older, natural women in their mid-fifties that resembled their early forties. Then one woman came on the show and I believe she was 58 and I swear she looked more youthful than I did at that time. Wow! What was her secret?

Preparation H

I want you to visualize a long-haired blonde that hopped in her big, black pickup truck speeding to the closest pharmacy store to buy this secret. Oh yes, I didn't hesitate. The proof was in the pudding. This woman looked remarkable and I knew from my early days of modeling that this had been used before for that tired, baggy-eyed look. But I had no idea that it worked for wrinkles, too.

So for the next couple of months while I was involved in promoting and selling the facial products that worked on a 'cellular level', I secretly began my own strategy. At night I covered my wrinkle spots with the Preparation H and in the daytime I would wear it under my face powder. During this time I had a good friend that was actually one of those friends that like to scrutinize my looks on a daily basis. Do you have a friend like that? You know, the type that has you primping an extra ten minutes in the mirror so you pass the scrutiny and the 'once over' with their eyes when you first meet them.

Well, I met my friend and she immediately said, "Wow, those products you have been selling really work! Your skin looks amazing."

"Thanks!" I felt like such a fraud you know. Promoting products for women in my neighborhood, while slathering on the Preparation H. How do you confess that one to someone? Well, I had to tell someone. This secret was much too good to contain.

I responded, "I haven't been using those products lately. Actually I have something to confess. I saw this *Oprah Winfrey Show*. I am using...

... Preparation H!"

Yes, a gasp did follow and, "Are you kidding me?"

My secret was out. Soon I had to say goodbye to the group of women and those products I would no longer use. I actually am one of those persons that must believe in what they are promoting.

You could say this secret eventually lead to my career in the newspaper business, which was much more fun anyway. I religiously kept this product with me through the years and boldly did confess to those that asked. That was in 2005. What happened when I ran out of Preparation H? Well, sometimes I would substitute Vaseline. Yes, that massive tub of petroleum slathering ointment we associate with babies and my mother's beauty cabinet products from the seventies… and was invented in *1872!*

An Oldie But Goodie

What I discovered is that Vaseline works just slightly better than my first discovery. And the best news is it's not as embarrassing to share with your friends like Preparation H. You can actually tell someone and they are not freaked out by your beauty secret. Although injecting Botulinum into your skin sounds pretty scary to me. So at least that was just a cream that had a specific use that worked.

Nowadays I personally prefer Vaseline with vitamin E. That's my top-notch secret that actually works against preempting the stages of deeper wrinkles. It works just as well and I have less shame in carrying it around in my handbag.

Now why again does this work? *Why?*

Because it keeps your skin super moist and petroleum is so thick it does not seep into your skin. It stays on top acting as a protective shield against the environment, dryness and those unwanted pillow wrinkles we all experience especially if you like to sleep on your side or on your stomach. If you can teach yourself to sleep on your back and stay there, well, then that's one more added trick that will keep your skin less wrinkled over the years.

So, do you share this secret with your friends?

Yes!

I have no idea why women like to keep beauty secrets from each other. Although I tend to have that 'too nice persona' that may make others think I am a sap for sharing such secrets. If you don't want to tell, you don't have to confess that you are benefiting from using plain old Vaseline from the Dollar Store.

I know. It somehow lacks that glamour that the fancy word 'Botox' has. It sure doesn't sound sexy does it? However, if it works, who cares?

My advice to you is try this for one week and see if you notice a difference. Life is too short to be frightened of slathering Vaseline across your crow's feet. Why not see if it can work for you, too?

I just read in a recent article that one of the *Friends'* stars shared in a magazine feature this is one of her simple secrets, too. I can give you a hint. She was the one that started a really cool hair trend and was by far my favorite character on the show. Now I love her as a woman for being one of those 'friends' that shares what works for her when it comes to looking fabulous over forty. After all, if you can't be a true friend and share your beauty secret, are you really friends with your friends? That's definitely something to ponder. After all, you only have one face. What to do? Protect it with one of the very first skin protectants ever invented… *Vaseline.* I do! Hey, don't just take my word for it. Do some semi-investigating online and actually give it a trial run for one week. You won't be disappointed. Especially when your once 'Reserve for Botox' money is now being used instead on spoiling your family with a fabulous vacation. That will feel so much more rewarding, too.

Chapter 29

Pressure to Feel Beautiful? Should We or Shouldn't We?

Does trying to be beautiful and the best you can possibly be mean that you are shallow and vain? Recently there has been speculation regarding this subject, especially for women that are mothers and approaching midlife. Why so much pressure to look good? Is it really necessary to glam it up, wear lipstick, be fashionable when you are running a household full of children, while maybe even working a nine to five job, too? Why throw added pressure onto the equation with our looks?

Legendary Estée Lauder once said:

Beauty is an attitude. There is no secret. Why are all brides beautiful? Because on their wedding day they care how they look. There are no ugly women. Only women that don't care or don't believe they are attractive.

You don't have to be a model in order to exude beauty. As I stated in the beginning, beauty is first a soulful journey. One must embrace themselves from the inside out in order to feel truly beautiful, even on the outside. My goal with this book is to inspire women that may not normally be motivated to take care of themselves because they feel they are middle aged and think, "What's the use?"

I want to change your attitude. There is no reason to throw in the towel at any age.

I recently just read an article about a woman that wrote a book regarding why she chose to stop trying to look good. She hung towels over mirrors and stopped wearing makeup. Her experiment was the extreme opposite of this book I guess. I say good for her. If that is what it took for her to get in touch with her soul and discover what really makes her tick from the inside out, that is what she needed to do.

My personal experience as a woman is to share with you that trying to look, feel and actually stay healthy will improve your own self-image over time. I went through one of those periods when I lived in braids and baggy sweatpants with nothing but some lipstick on. I don't think it is a coincidence now when looking back that this was one of the humdrum times of my life. While I had taken on that self-martyr role of 'being a mother and running the household, don't I do so much already why try' attitude, I can tell you I had definitely lost that certain something that gave me the confidence of my twenties. I remember thinking, "This must just be the stages of life. Now I am older and those things are really not important anymore."

Wrong.

I had just moved from the crazy pace of Los Angeles and moved into an affluent community that consisted of golf courses and Tuscany-style homes. I didn't see the point in trying to look fabulous in this new environment. What's the point of this? Who cares what I look like anyway?

That was until I met a new friend that was absolutely gorgeous and had that kind of persona that made you want to look fabulous, too. She sparkled at the Gymboree mom groups. Her hair looked shiny. Her face had some rouge. How refreshing it was to see a woman trying to look fabulous even though they were driving an SUV soccer mom's vehicle.

Well, my new friendship inspired me. I began fixing my hair again. Soon I stopped braiding my hair and wore more of a Darryl Hannah *Splash* look. I found my old Levi's and bought some colorful blouses that revealed my natural figure. I stopped running around like a lifeless zombie. I added some pizzazz back into my daily attire. I had connected again with just a touch of glamour that reminded me that it feels rewarding to look good.

So for me personally to just *throw in the towel* is like covering up a mirror on my favorite part of being a woman… which is what? I can dress up and express my soul from the inside out! I can feel feminine and beautiful with simple steps that do not require me to spend hours in front of the mirror. A little effort applied at the beginning of the day added that extra step and smile I had been missing. Why not try it for yourself, too?

From that period on, I have never been one of those moms that doesn't wear makeup. For my soul, that just doesn't work. I happen to feel brighter from the inside out by caring enough to make an effort with my appearance.

There is no reason to dislike celebrities for being glamorous and beautiful.

Be your own celebrity. Uncover your mirrors in your home. Take time to like your face, accentuate it and add some lipstick to your natural lips. Wear simple jewelry. Invest in some basics for your wardrobe that you feel confident in which can be dressed up or down by changing a blouse or a skirt. You can buy clothes from upscale consignment shops that cut the cost of shopping. This still happens to be my favorite way to save money. If I never told anyone, most wouldn't know that my Cavalli T-shirt was only ten dollars. If you don't have extra money right now to do a little shopping, clean out your closet and organize it. Create some outfits from what you already have hanging in the closet.

Try to be stylish and care about how you look because after all, why would you not want to be the best you can be? Life is too short to sell ourselves excuses like now we are older so let's cut ourselves some slack.

Madonna is Madonna because she has dedicated her life to caring about her outer appearance and does not let society's judgment ever negate her style and clothing. She's not concerned whether or not she can wear a short skirt because she is over fifty.

She just wears what she wants to whenever she wants. Yes, she is Madonna. But you can be bold, too, in your own world.

You can make yourself and your own natural beauty a priority.

Why not try and look like a superstar? Imitate the greats. Take time and like yourself and enhance your natural beauty. Invest in you as you would others in your world. Trust me, I still have a pajama day. I allow myself one of those days to just unwind with no makeup on and I just curl up by the fire and read a book.

Okay, I will admit it. I am guilty of once in awhile running an errand in my flannel pajamas when I have run out of coffee creamer at home. I have been the mother wearing a baggy trench coat over her flannel pajamas with Ugg slippers on. But...

Don't you just hate when you see that someone special or someone you haven't seen in awhile and they catch you in your pajamas at the supermarket? I do. I try very hard to cut those moments down to a minimum. *I make some time for me before I leave the house.*

So don't leave the house without looking your best because you never know what opportunity might be lurking around the corner. You don't want to miss out on the unexpected 'life-changing moment' because you were too lazy to find some style and apply a dab of lipstick. It doesn't take much to spruce up, even just a little. So don't be a martyr as a woman. Don't make excuses because of your tasks. Be prepared. Face the world with your best foot forward and take pride in your looks and beauty.

Life can be brutal. So look beautiful.

Make time each day for a little style and makeup. Ask yourself, what statement do you want to make today? Embrace your best and be your best. For those of you that would rather just sit on the couch, eating bonbons and watching those real housewives in some neighborhood, take my advice and become your own star. Get creative and be somebody in your own world. Spend a little more time and devotion toward *yourself*. Forsake pity. Become hip and beautiful.

After all, why should Madonna get to be the only rock star? There is no reason to ever throw in the towel because of age. Remember there is only one you. So do your best to look your best. Why? Because *you* deserve it!

Chapter 30

What is Your Weekly Beauty Regimen?

When I was fifteen years old I spent my extra time at a modeling school learning how to present myself, take care of my skin and what *not* to do. One little secret I learned was never use your index finger to remove makeup off of your eyelids. Why? Because you will apply too much force over many years of doing this and cause your skin to sag faster by your own beauty habit. Ouch. What to do instead? Use your wedding finger (the closest one to your small finger) because it uses the least amount of pressure.

I learned to wash my face every day and every night with a three-step method:

- Soap/cleanser product
- Toner
- Moisturizer

I remember encountering friends and women in my early twenties that would not wash their face before they went to sleep. I would secretly worry about their face breaking out and desperately wanted to tell them the importance of a simple beauty routine every night. What I have discovered over the decades of friends from all ages, is that because I was a model at an early age I became privy to some information that others might have missed. If you were not reading *Cosmopolitan* or *Mademoiselle* then these are basic steps you might skip.

A simple doable beauty regimen is absolutely imperative on your road to Middle Age Beauty. If you have sort of neglected this off and on in your life, there is no time like the present to start today.

Each night before you go to bed:

Remove makeup from your face with a product that you find works well. I know everyone has a different skin type, so what works for me may not work well for you. I happen to love Burt's Bees facial soap, Pond's Cold Cream or even just Noxzema.

Next follow up with a toner. I happen to like the Oxy Pads which happen to clean the dirt you might have missed without that second step.

Moisturizer... Yes! This is absolutely important, especially during our Middle Age Beauty years. Keeping your skin moist and soft combats natural dryness and helps slow down the wrinkle process. Do take time and find a great moisturizer that works for you. I will let you know in one of my next chapters the best ones I have found that you can also buy for yourself, too. You don't need to spend over a hundred dollars on a cream when you can find the same ones within reach with the same ingredients.

In the Morning: Wash your face lightly again and then apply sunscreen. I use an SPF 15 sunscreen by Oil of Olay. This works wonderfully and does not clog up my pores or make my face feel greasy. You may need to select a different product that will be better for you.

The Mini-Spa Day: Yes, that's right. Once a week I have my own mini-spa day where I devote one long hour to an indulging soak in my bathtub. I light a candle and close my eyes and relax to the sound of... nothing. I condition my hair for a few minutes with an over-the-counter conditioner, then cover myself in mint julep mud mask, which helps shrink the appearance of your pores.

I respect my body and soul once a week by unwinding from the hectic pace. How? By rejuvenating my skin, hair, and body. I even do some of those deep breathing exercises I mentioned in the Soul section. I consciously choose to book a date with myself once a week, which helps me remember to love myself, care for myself and to baby my body with love.

This little mini-spa day always adds that something extra for me to look forward to the following weekend. Many times we feel we have to travel or visit a spa to find some relaxation. Really we just have to make a strenuous effort to become creative and make our lives a little more exciting and beautiful. Make time for your beauty regimen each week. Soon you won't even think about it, and it will become part of your daily schedule. Don't skip out on the basics. But do skip out on those needles at the medical spa. Those are not necessary if you are managing your time and yourself wisely. *OK?*

Chapter 31

Nature Hikes Help You Connect with Your Inner Beauty

In order to stay beautiful and healthy these days, there are all sorts of angles on how to do it. The one you will not find in this book is using a plastic surgeon to maintain a youthful appearance. You can try yoga. You can try spinning. You can find a hypnotist that helps you relax your years away from adding age to your skin. You can use expensive creams. You can try getting extra sleep. However, there is nothing like taking a walk in nature to connect with your soul. Remember at the beginning of this book one of the most important 'Dos' is to experience three acts of joy a day.

Connecting to your soul and prying your mind away from the hectic stress of life is an option we often forget to exercise quite figuratively speaking. I found that hiking in the area where I live has given my workout routine a pleasant adjustment. No longer do I just run in my neighborhood out of convenience; I also force myself to take advantage of the abundance of hiking trails in Southern California.

How does this connect to beauty versus health? Nature hikes allow me to connect with part of myself that I cannot always access. The quietness of the trail, the peaceful getaway from the city instantly relaxes my face. My worries are temporarily forgotten as I begin to observe and appreciate the different colors of green foliage or how the sunlight is casting shadows across the hillsides. I recognize the blue sky and observe its texture in the way it hits the horizon. I gaze into nature and suddenly forget the immediacy of tasks and daily pressures.

This weekly retreat has become one of my small joys each week that allows me to find that inner calm and serenity that I sometimes have trouble finding in California. When I am relaxed, my face relaxes. I find a balance between myself and the essence of nature surrounding me. This balance adds to my beauty equation. These hikes have added something extra I had been currently missing up until the beginning of this year.

I suggest that you can take a break and discover nature walks in the areas where you live. Maybe you live in New York and Central Park is your escape. Maybe you live in Florida and you prefer walks on the beach. The important factor is submerging your soul with the peace and serenity that nature offers us free of charge. Seek refuge in the rolling waves on a sandy beach, take a stroll by the lakes or creeks near your home.

When I lived in Los Angeles, I found my reprieve from society running around Lake Hollywood, a reservoir not too far from where I lived. My point is, if you search you can find your moments of peace maybe even within reach of your front door. Are you making time to discover the beauty of nature? Nature in turn reminds us to look within and search for beauty within ourselves. As Audrey Hepburn stated, beauty is not in a facial mode, and something we carry within ourselves and display for the rest of the world to see. There is nothing wrong with trying to strive for outer beauty.

What we present to the world is up to us

How we find the means to look our best can sometimes require us to become resourceful and discover the healing power of nature and why it's essential for our health, mind and soul.

The benefits of Connecting to Nature:

Quieting your mind.
Connecting to the energy of the earth, and its natural habitat allows for body renewal and mind renewal.
Walking in calming surroundings helps alleviate stress.
Helps fight the 'moody blues' and depression.

The act of walking outside during the daylight hours helps us receive that hour of light exposure we should be getting once a day for our vitamin D source.

Beauty is ultimately a choice. You can choose to strive for your natural right to feel beautiful from the inside out by actively seeking ways to improve your mental and physical health. I know that my Midwestern roots have lent to my constant search of connecting to nature over the many different chapters of my life. I count myself lucky for learning at an early age why 'the great outdoors' can be many things to us, including a fabulous retreat. Your mood and energy will also improve from seeking this quiet solace each week from nature.

Make a point to add to your list each week. Rain, snow or sunshine, embrace the beauty that God has given each of us to benefit from each day.

I do suggest if it's below freezing temperatures to wait for a warmer day. I suggest always alerting those you know to where you will be if you are going on a nature hike alone. Take your dog with you if you have one. Invest in a small pepper spray and learn how to use it. Never risk your safety for the sake of peace or beauty. Walk with a friend if you can or walk in areas that are safe. Do a little research before you go hiking in an area you have never gone before. Be cognizant of your surroundings. I personally never walk on the trails on the same day or time. I constantly change my routine just in case someone could be watching. I hate to weave in such a scare tactic here, but I just want you to think wisely before you go off into the woods alone. Connecting to nature can also be as simple as taking a stroll in your neighborhood.

Chapter 32

ICON Chic

Audrey Hepburn died January 20, 1993. I remember when I heard the news. I was standing at a gas station in downtown Kansas City near the Plaza at nighttime talking to my mother on the payphone.

"Have you heard?" Mom asked.

"What?" I asked her back, instinctively knowing that it would not be good news.

"Audrey Hepburn died today."

I stood there in the chilly cold night as a young woman with my life before me. I just found out the most shattering fact. The woman that I adored had left this earth. I wept softly. I felt like I had missed an opportunity of connecting with her. I had just moved to California only couple of years before. Even though she lived in Switzerland, I had the fantastic dream that I might somehow run into her when she came to Los Angeles for an event. Her grace, her movies, her natural looks and contribution to fight hunger as head of UNICEF inspired me as a young woman to try to become something 'real' versus plastic as a person.

This goal truly had its limitations when you were a model and lived in Hollywood.

Hoping to be 'real' in a world where my modeling Zed Card displayed photos and statistics that included: Height, Weight, Bust Size, Hips and my age clearly told another story than one of substance. I sat in lines with other girls at 'Go-Sees', hoping to land modeling work with these numbers that categorized me as a 'Face and Lingerie model' versus high fashion. I learned tips as a model that helped conceal pimples, and weight loss tips about eating apples and only water before a swimsuit photo shoot. I worried constantly about what I ate, if my hair was long enough, if my shoes were fashionable, how others perceived my beauty. I also became worried about an expiration date in the fashion industry. At the age of twenty years old, I already felt like a 'has-been' and knew the clock was ticking on how many more bookings could be mine before I became too old to be a model.

I worked steadily as a model booking in smaller markets like San Francisco and then on to Los Angeles. By the time Audrey Hepburn died, my heart had hardened toward the strictness of the modeling business. My soul felt incomplete by the mere nature of how the business was truly superficial. Shortly after Audrey's death, an unusual moment occurred. After having a disagreement with a booker at Elite in Los Angeles, my words surprised me: "Just throw my portfolio in the trash! I'm done with this business."

"Really." I had heard a gasp at the other end of the phone, then silence.

Okay. That was that, I remember thinking.

But this was not the end of my career as a model. I continued to book work later on. Commercials and modeling are so inter-twined; there was no way around it. Honestly, there is a thin line between the two. The only real acting I had ever done ended in an art house film and a few bit parts on sitcoms and improv days in comedy. Eventually at the age of 27 after booking several commercials and working as an actress, I landed a serious face ad campaign with St. Ives Apricot Scrub. With my face plastered throughout *Cosmopolitan*, *Good Housekeeping* and many other magazines you would think that I would have been strolling through the airports that year beaming with pride and a sense of accomplishment with tearing out my own piece of success in both industries. Instead, I began to feel a deep inner sense of sadness that could not be filled by my face glowing in an orange hue stuck between the pages of other model 'tear sheets'. My achievement as a model or a working actress felt numbered and meaningless if it could all just end with the blossom of youth fading with the time. Could this have been an early midlife crisis about turning thirty shortly? The feeling of sorrow stayed with me. How can I be worth anything if age will keep on robbing me of the things I naturally wanted in my career?

When life gives us unexpected circumstances that we have never planned on, it's up to us to dig deeper to find out what *we* can do about fixing what could be wrong.

Raised by two upbeat parents, that regularly said, "Life's short, so be happy," I did not feel good about these feelings of inadequacy. I had been taught to not pity myself and to make the most of what I have now.

So I went in search of help. I found out about a 'Life Coach' through a friend of mine like I mentioned earlier. A Zen spiritual teacher that revealed insightful, deeper lessons the 'surface world of modeling and acting' could not reveal to me. A third party that played a significant role was my grandmother. Grandma Lula would send me Norman Vincent Peale pamphlets in the mail almost weekly. With this three-step approach of finding out and exploring my inner feelings, I discovered there was more to life than my measurements, my face and what others perceived of me. I managed to break out of that shallow mold of 'surface' thinking and find more meaningful blessings that came from within my soul.

Shortly after working through this inner turmoil of uncertainty, my 'life turned the corner', as they say. I became certain about who I was on the inside and new exciting things evolved. I joined the writer's program at UCLA; a play I had written was chosen by the HBO Workspace to be showcased, which I produced, directed and starred in as the leading actress. I had finally found my footing…

Until the age of 39, that is. You guessed it. That expiration date had arrived again. That dreaded 4-0 was only weeks away. I wanted desperately to keep living, except without *those* digits attached. You know, the one with the list of desperate housewives on reality shows, soccer moms, cougars, fillers, implants, and the countless list of needle injections that were recommended if you actually stepped foot into a medical spa. I did not want to become that woman.

Now living near Rancho Santa Fe, an affluent enclave of San Diego, you can only guess the insane need of trying to stay young and buxom in Southern California. While others bragged openly about their Botox treatments, Audrey Hepburn and my Grandma Lula would always pop into my mind.

What would Audrey think? Would Grandma approve of Botox?

Those two lucid questions kept me digging into my own medicine cabinet for my own antidote of skin care creams, some under one dollar. Trust me, this is not a fact you would like to brag about in the world full of sunny weather, Bentleys and Yves Saint Laurent. I kept my secrets well intact!

When my big 4-0 only was weeks away, at least my writing career had wings as well. Working for a couple of community newspapers, I slowly built my 'by lines' and found my way into the hearts of readers as a columnist writing about the local socialites in the ritzy area. On occasion I would write about my thoughts, too. Including why I had chosen my grandmother's approval over Botulism injections.

So back to the meltdown, the dreaded dead, black roses and all of the 'over the hill' jokes. I could not escape *that* number.

As you know from my letter in the beginning, I woke up feeling exuberantly happy, which frankly was quite shocking after fretting about this age thing for so many years.

I didn't *feel* any different. I managed to climb into a new decade. With this thought arriving in my head, I realized overall I had found something unique due to some early lessons that lead me into my middle-aged experience with an excellent foundation full of youth and promise.

Now back to that young girl crying in the phone booth in a rainstorm. Yes, Audrey Hepburn had left this planet that day, but her spirit and grace has lived on through all of her movies, pictures and her dedication to making this world a more beautiful place by helping others.

During my soul searching, I had found an Icon to inspire me with beauty, elegance and style. I copied Audrey's glasses. I wore dresses that looked like hers and found jackets that helped me conquer a room with confidence just because I stood in the door in a well-tailored coat. Audrey Hepburn helped inspire me to find my own style in the beginning of my 'womanhood'.

I went through a phase where I read every book on Audrey. I collected her movies. I had almost everyone one of them. One of my prized possessions still to this day is of an original movie poster of Audrey Hepburn's movie *Two for the Road*. Her smile always looked bright and curious. Her eyes sparkled with enthusiasm. I wanted to emulate those things, too. I liked her effervescent spirit.

Do you have an Icon?

Have you had challenging times in your life when your age confined your thinking? If you can find an Icon that can inspire you while giving you inspiration in style, this can help you break that cycle that we as women can fall into when we start obsessing on our age.

One of the other things I admired dearly about Audrey was her natural beauty. Absolutely natural. She aged with dignity and grace and still had that ingénue quality that never left her. She was forever youthful at heart.

So here is your assignment. If you don't have an Icon, find one today. Find someone that you admire as a person for their style, life and any other assets that can help you benefit from learning from their example.

At any point on our journey, we may need a teacher to teach us things. An Icon you may never meet, but you can learn from watching and studying them from afar, too. A mentor and an Icon is always important to find. In the process, you can become your own Icon. *Be bold, and don't be held back by a number.*

Chapter 33

Think PINK!

What you wear affects your mood. Have you noticed that? For most of my life I have been one of those women that embrace that New York chic look wearing black in many facets of my life. Because I am blonde I have always felt that I look like cotton candy at the fair during the hot weather in summer. Well, that's how I felt. Then a few years back as I was driving my son to school he asked me, "Mom, why do you always wear black?" I replied to him, "Because I like it I guess. "But, Mom, you always wear black." My son had a good point. Who wants to be predictable. Who wants to be one of those persons that someone can guess what they will wear every day?

Since this conversation and also because my husband prefers it when I wear color, I have begun to branch out and wear colors more often. I found that greens work well for me, some softer yellows and reds. I will buy scarves with a splash of color to add to my current black wardrobe. For example, even today as I was getting ready to go to work with my husband at his shop (I always wear my workout clothes because there are these fabulous hiking trails behind his family's business) I had once again fallen into my trap of wearing black. Black shorts, black tank top and oh so boring. I remembered that indeed to feel a little more cheerful is to add color, so I changed into a blue workout tank shirt instead. Immediately my mood felt less dreary and serious. The color I was wearing had indeed influenced my mood.

Are you like me and you tend to dress in the same colors all the time? Do yourself a favor and change it up. Our mood and our energy are the lifeline to how we function during the day. Just like I said about adding glamour to your look before you leave the house, you need to do the same with your clothes. Over the last four years I have added many color choices to my wardrobe. The change has not only affected how I feel, but also these colors can inspire my evening to feel more carefree, and not be so severely dressed in black all of the time.

Think about all of the colors you see on the shows geared toward women today. From Manhattan to Miami, these women are wearing bright vibrant colors that give their aura a more youthful appearance. I will confess to you that black just happens to be that one choice in my wardrobe that can build my confidence like no other, so I do tend to lean on that for an important interview in which I feel I can muster my best foot forward. However, what I do now is add a touch of color somewhere in my outfit. For example if I wear a corporate-looking black tailored jacket, I wear underneath it a vibrant pink color that 'pops' from underneath. I don't just wear only from 'head to toe' black. It's amazing how much more bold and carefree I feel with that little something extra that can add the zest and excitement, and in turn improve my mood. Think back to when we were all children. Remember how inspiring it was to have those pink colors in our rooms, to pink notepads, hot pink erasers to the bubble gum in the hot colorful wrappers?

This chapter is entitled "Think Pink" for a reason.

Pink just happens to be my favorite color that brings out my playful side and inspires me to lighten up on my feet. I have a special set of pink flannel pajamas reserved for my cozy nights at home when I am able to indulge in a guilty pleasure by the fire and watch *Celebrity Ghost Stories*. I have a pink jacket, a pink sweater, and pink workout long-sleeve shirts that immediately shave off a few years from my appearance because I am wearing youthful colors.

Don't buy into that philosophy that now you are older and you have to dress more maturely. Do you think Madonna is thinking that? Do you want to be a matronly woman that seems too conservative because you are wearing clothes you *think* you should be wearing because of your age? Don't be fooled by what you think is appropriate, go by what's in your soul. I never realized the impact of colors on my mood until I began changing up my style. So take my advice and go back to your childhood and unleash your favorite color in your mind. Now start adding it in your daily ritual somewhere, like maybe it's a purse, a new phone cover, or a new shawl that you can take and drape around your shoulders. Your favorite color will bring back some of those spunky feelings we sometimes feel we have to lose now because we are adults. If you want to live a full and vibrant life, don't do what I did and wear only black. The reason there is a saying "From out of the mouth of babes" is because it is true.

Did you know in ancient times in China and Egypt, they practiced what they called 'chromotherapy', which was the practice of using colors to heal a patient's health. This practice is still used today as an alternative or holistic treatment. Maybe I love pink because it's associated with love and romance. Pink is also known as a calming color, which works well with my fast-paced personality. It's good for me to find that grounding and brings me back to my little girl self that needs to be nurtured.

According to a recent survey undertaken in the UK, researchers also found that wearing tighter and trendier clothes could shave off fifteen years. One of their recommendations found in this article was to avoid washed out and drab colors. (I do think my son knew what he was talking about!) This study showed that adding a bold color statement came in at the top of the list. Other tips included wearing a bra that fits you well with excellent support and wearing trendy clothes that fit your body well help shave off the years. Wearing baggy and an undistinguished style is the first thing that needs to go. So back to the other chapter on why appearance matters, remember that color matters, too.

Why spend your hard-earned money on controversial facial treatments when you can instead learn how to become creative by adding bolder colors and trendier styles to your wardrobe? Don't be fooled. Yes, you may be middle-aged, but that doesn't mean you need to resort to drastic measures by adding crazy fillers to your face. And, think of all of the fun you can have by reinventing yourself with little splashes of color mixed in to your daily to-do list? Maybe you already have that color thing mastered, but this was definitely one that I learned during my mid-thirties thanks to my son's honest opinion of my style one day on our way to school together. His foresight has had an impact on my mood, my closet and most of all my appearance.

Here are some of my suggestions to you that have helped me spruce up my wardrobe with inexpensive touches over the last few years:

- Figure out what your favorite color was as a child. Now begin to add that color to your daily life. This could even be a coffee mug you carry every day at work. I have vamped up my purse by adding a pink Kenneth Cole wallet and a glitzy pink phone case. I'm not living in New York. So I don't need to dress like I work in a museum.
- Buy some interchangeable scarves and shawls that you can take on the go. Drape a scarf around your neck or carry it with you for a little flair. Be exotic and add some flowing material to your day. Yes, I am even talking to those of you with little babies that think you need to be more pragmatic. You have the right to look and feel gorgeous, too.
- Buy a selection of T-shirts or blouses that you can wear and interchange with other styles in your wardrobe. This extra touch of color will give you a youthful and more flattering appearance without breaking your wallet.
- Add your color to your accessories like a purse, a belt, a wallet or some eye-popping jewelry. (I know scarves could

fit here, but they are such a fashion statement they deserve their own merit!)

- Don't forget your nails and your toes. Always keep those looking bright and beautiful.

Once I went to a golf event with some friends to attend a ritzy dinner. At the end of the evening one of the football players told me all of the guys were secretly polling which girl had the best pedicure. Can you believe it, I won? When I told him, I just do them myself, he walked away looking a little shocked and fooled. Hey, girls, the trick is to just place a little effort into our lives because we never know who we might meet or who might be scrutinizing our feet at the end of the day!

Remember to think pink and add your own color to your life. This isn't a dress rehearsal. So take some time and figure out how to enhance your journey with simple changes that can influence your mood and the world around you. Be creative with color when it comes to expressing yourself. One of my favorite quotes ever is by my personal favorite icon, Audrey Hepburn. She also embraced pink as a color to love. Here are her lovely thoughts to add sparkle to your day:

"I believe in pink. I believe that laughing is the best calorie burner. I believe in kissing, kissing a lot. I believe in being strong when everything seems to be going wrong. I believe that happy girls are the prettiest girls. I believe that tomorrow is another day and I believe in miracles."

Chapter 34

Keep Fashion Simple

I think I mentioned how when I arrived in San Francisco, my modeling agent helped me discover fashion. What you may not believe is even though it was over 22 years ago, most of her advice still holds true to today's fashion standards.

So here they are, those simple rules that will help you add easy chic to your wardrobe with a simple style:

- Black jeans/solid dark blue jeans.
- T-shirts with color. Bold colors along with one white one and a black one.
- A good pair of walking boots. Do think Nancy Sinatra here.
- Trendy long and short jackets. Think wraparound black New York style and a simple basic blue denim jean jacket.
- Earrings – keep them simple. (Please don't mimic the reality show women.)
- One black go-see dress. Or that classic Audrey Hepburn *Breakfast at Tiffany's* style.
- Heels – Add comfortable heels to your wardrobe. Making yourself taller is also slenderizing.
- Headband. You know like the one Bridget Bardot used to wear? A perfect accessory to create that chic statement.
- Belts and handbags. Have at least one killer belt and one amazing handbag that you can sling over your shoulder that makes you feel like a sexy woman.
- Black leggings (recently made a comeback!).

Okay, that was the list. Nothing extravagant. Nothing too trendy and everything mentioned are still current trends today. Sometimes wearing too much clothing that looks like Cleopatra is trendy, but does the style look right for your body shape?

Also, before you get into those skinny black leggings, do turn around and check yourself in the mirror. Sometimes leggings are too thin and can show a little too much skin in the daylight if you are not covering it up.

Miniskirts that are not too mini are also important to keep in our wardrobe. Don't listen to those naysayers that will tell you are too old to wear a mini-skirt. Just make sure it's not too short and your legs do look fabulous enough to show them. Nothing looks better than a pair of black go-go boots with a trendy mini-skirt. Don't forget you do want to turn some heads as you are arriving at work or even meeting your mom's group out at Starbucks. Be bold and try to look chic every day, too. Sometimes simplicity is the key to everything, isn't it?

So remember, don't always get caught up in the fads. Rely on some basic classics that you can mix and match easily into your already existing wardrobe. Coordinate the outfits. Always set your outfit next to your bed so you can be ready to tackle your new day with confidence and ease.

One of the worst feelings for me is when I am running late and I am still anxiously trying on an assortment of tops because I didn't make time the night before.

A big part of the beauty equation if you haven't noticed by now is order and planning.

Plan ahead. Get enough sleep, make time for joyful moments, create prizefighting Rocky Like Moments and so on. In order to create the world we wish we could have, all we need to do *now* is become organized enough to manifest it. Life can still be spontaneous, but only in a *Harry Met Sally* kind of Meg Ryan way, like when you are having a fun conversation at the deli and you want to drive home a point to a good friend.

Chapter 35

Beauty Product Tips

(Please note, if you can not find these in your personal neighborhood, all of these products can be purchased online for similar pricing.)

I've already shared with you my ultimate wrinkle secret that is as simple as Vaseline. You might be chuckling at that line but until you try it consecutively for a few days you will never know the benefits of this product that even our grandmothers used. Known as a skin protectant, those four words alone should do the trick in at least steering you away from the Botox clique in your neighborhood. I love the friends that have a good laugh behind my back regarding this tip.

I just want to reiterate an extremely important point before I share a few more products that you can use and like, too. This book isn't really about beauty tips as it's more about taking simple measures to help simplify your life. When we simplify those things that surround us, we can find an inner peace and calm from within. Going within and connecting with the 'inner you' is the number one goal of *Middle Age Beauty*. To help redirect your steps to your inside first before finding and criticizing ourselves.

It can be so challenging to be a woman these days. From maybe working two jobs, to feeding children, planning meals, keeping a house clean... where do you find time for you?

Remember you have to schedule the moments in. Become a little more organized for moments with yourself. If that means walking on the beach once this week or meeting a friend for a coffee, schedule it in!

Yesterday I drove up to Los Angeles to meet a great friend of mine. In order to plan that day and have the most glowing positive experience, I chose to commit. I managed to make it work with my family and made it happen. We must plan ahead in order to see the results we are at least expecting to happen.

Driving in bumper-to-bumper traffic from San Diego to Los Angeles could've have been one factor that might have prevented me from experiencing this amazing day. However, sometimes we must press on through difficult obstacles in order to create our bliss.

When I arrived at the Conscious Life Expo at the LAX Hilton Hotel, I quickly changed out of my sweats and into a more tailored look for the event. I wore a long skirt with leopard matching heels and jacket. Nothing overtly glamorous, but I will admit I did feel rather smartly dressed for the event. As I have said before, what you wear matters. Clothes can make you feel like a million dollars. You don't have to be rich to know how to shop. You just have to make a little effort. So what is the purpose of bringing up this day?

Well, I stepped off my regular schedule to do something enriching for my soul. In turn, that night I slept better. I felt more relaxed and at ease in my own skin.

What happens when we Experience moments of Inner Peace?

Our face muscles relax. Our worry lines cease. We take deeper breaths. The more balance we feel inside, the less stressed we feel. What can stress do? Cause wrinkles.

So remember if you have skipped ahead to the beauty section, make sure you go back and read the Soul section next. Because that's the essence of 'you'. What you feel in your inner world will definitely reflect on your expression. So please know that making peace with your inner world is so important. Learn to love you. Learn to be kinder and nicer to yourself each day. And the rest of these beauty products are more like the finishing touches that we can apply with a last minute thought because we are taking time to take care of ourselves on the 'inside, too'.

Skin care: The most important thing to know regarding your skin care is that you should absolutely take time moisturizing and washing your face properly every day. I can count on my hands how many times I have gone to sleep with makeup on my face, and it's not too many. The key to good skin is to keep it clean, fresh and moisturized and protected.

Sunblock – $8.50 to $16.00 Oil of Olay Daily UV Moisturizer: Please remember each person has an issue that may differ from mine. For example, I personally have to watch the dark spots since I have a fair complexion. So every day I use sunblock in the morning. Don't think that heavy 70 SPF type you wear in the summertime. Think light and not too oily. I personally like Oil of Olay's Daily UV Moisturizer. Don't forget to place this on your neck and the top of your chest, too. Your neck always needs to be included in your moisturizing area. This may be your most important tip here in this book. I know you have heard to always wear sunblock. So don't ignore this suggestion. Every little measure we take helps us retain that youthful, young skin that does need protecting from the sun.

**Wear makeup over your sunblock, too. That also acts as one more layer which protects the skin throughout the day.

Moisturizers that aid in skin and wrinkle repair: Well, just like you I have tried many. So just know the one I am recommending is one that I absolutely love the best. This product you may have to buy online or at a beauty store. But don't worry, you will be happy when it arrives at your doorstep. Shopping online at Amazon can be a rewarding experience.

Stretch Mark Complex – price $17.49 to $19.99: This product comes in right around the $20.00 mark. But compared to other stretch mark creams that can be as costly as $100.00, this is inexpensive. Don't let the name fool you. This can be used for a moisturizer for your face and is an intense moisturizing cream that nourishes your skin. Whenever I run out, I am tempted to just go without just because it's not as easy to find like other skin cream choices. Then, within a few days, my skin feels less fresh and more on the dry side. I always end up buying it immediately. This is my favorite moisturizer to date. This product improves the texture of your skin. Your face just feels like silk after applying it. I use it at nighttime and in the morning before I apply my sunblock. Remember the elements out there can chisel rocks, so make sure you are properly shielded with proper moisturizer every day. (Great reviews online, too.)

How I made the discovery? My mother. She called me up and told me she had been using this new cream from the beauty supply store. Then she shipped one to me in the mail and it's my absolute must-have right next to my tub of Vaseline inside my medicine cabinet, neatly aligned next to the sunblock.

Burt's Bees Radiance Night Cream – price $17.99: My second choice that you can find at your local pharmacy. This is an excellent second choice that works almost as well. The reviews are excellent online for this product, too. One woman wrote that it works better than most products she has tried costing hundreds of dollars. I agree with her because I have tried expensive creams, too. How I made the discovery? I found this one at a health food store near my house four years ago and liked it far better than an expensive one I was previously using.

Dark Spot Corrector – Porcelana Skin Lightening Cream – price $4.99: Active ingredient: 2% hydroquinone. (Recognized by the FDA as an effective product fighting against skin discoloration.) This product carries the same ingredient as many other expensive skin care lines with the same ingredient. Dark Spot Correctors can be anywhere from $60.00 dollars and up. So this product for me was an excellent find! I recommend using Porcelana if you have uneven tones or brown spots that can sometimes be too prevalent to your liking. Ask me, I know. Luckily for me though, I found this smart product that works well. It is suggested if you use the product to try and apply twice a day. I have noticed with more consistency, this product does indeed achieve the results you need.

How did I make this discovery? I went in search of this product since I am prone to dark spots with my fair complexion. I just happened to be lucky and found it right under my nose at the pharmacy.

Until you use a product for awhile, it's hard to know if it's working well. I can tell you I have used this product for almost two years. You will always find it in my medicine cabinet!

Mud Masks – Wrinkle reducer and helps prevent acne – $4.50– $8.00. Mint Julep Mud Masque by Queen Helene: Buy online or at a beauty supply store. (This is my secret that I have been using for years!)

Second choice: Freeman Clay Mask Avocado & Oatmeal Mask: Buy at the pharmacy. Once a week you can find me lounging in my home with a good book and a towel wrapped tightly around my hair, while wearing a neon green mud mask. I have been a big fan of mud masks for over twenty years. Maybe it's the association in my own mind, but I feel as if I am having my own spa day once a week in my own home. During my twenties I had one girlfriend ask me when we were hanging out at her apartment as I was resting with a mud mask, while she was doing her nails, why I liked those mud masks.

"Why do you do that so much to your skin?"

"I like them."

"Why?" she asked.

"I feel like I am in a mini-retreat!"

"Well," she responded, "I'm not so sure they are that good for your skin."

"Quite the contrary," I replied. Then we went back to our own thoughts and she finished her nails, as I closed my eyes, as my face grew tight from the crusted-over mask covering every inch of my face.

I have noticed since then there seems to be a myth some

associate with a mud mask that it dries out your skin and can age you. The facts are just the opposite. Besides making me feel relaxed, the main reason I wear them is because they are anti-aging and help reduce any problems with acne or blemishes, since acne can be triggered by oily skin. The tightening of the mask actually relaxes the muscles in your face. No wonder I feel like I am on a mini-retreat. Every worry line is relaxed as I sit back and take time to 'make time' to rejuvenate myself. This is a tip I definitely learned as a model. One of those tips that have stuck with me for a lifetime. Just remember like everything in life, use a mud mask in moderation. I wouldn't use it more than once a week. That happens to be my lucky number with it anyway.

Instant Tanning Cream – L'Oréal Sublime Bronze *medium, natural tan* – **$8.49:** You may not need this tip. You may have more of that olive, dark skin that looks always sunny and warm. I, however, am very pale naturally. So the trick is that I use this product the *day before* an important event or luncheon with my friends. Now I don't want you to think this makes you orange. Absolutely not. Instant tanning products have come a long way over the years. Now you can find many that work well, don't streak and give your skin tone the appearance of looking like you've been kissed by the sun. I only use this product on my arms, chest area and my legs. Do make sure to rinse your hands well with soap after applying. Also another easy trick is to add regular skin care moisturizer over it to make sure it's been applied evenly. This product also contains vitamin E, which is soothing to your skin. How I discovered this product? Neutrogena had stopped making one of my favorite tanning products and this proved to be the next best option.

Hair – Keratin Hair Treatment – Renpure Originals Brazilian Keratin 14 Day Straight Treatment – $5.99–$8.99: Do you remember how luxurious and gorgeous all of the *Friends* actresses' hair just looked – simply healthy and always beautiful?

Well, like other actresses in Hollywood, they were privy to a new treatment hitting America before the regular folks like us were able to find these products on the streets. Well, now we, too, can have gorgeous, healthy hair.

Okay, I know talking product talk isn't the most exciting thing, but when you struggle with naturally dry hair, this one tip is like finding the fountain of youth. Well, that's an exaggeration, but that is exactly how I felt the first time I went in for a professional Brazilian Blowout. I soon did some investigating and realized I could also give myself this exact treatment. The key to these products is that they are 'sulfate-free'. So I recommend the Renpure Originals. I now have much healthier hair. If you don't like having straight hair, you can always wash your hair at night and sleep with it in a loosely wrapped bun overnight. When you wake up just undo the bun and watch your hair look bouncy and beautiful.

These are my product tips for you. Try them. They have worked well for me. These are easy to find, simple solutions that can help you in your quest to look your best on your journey through your Middle Age Beauty years.

Like Thomas Moore suggested in *Care for the Soul*:

Tending the things around us and becoming more sensitive to importance of home, daily schedule, and maybe even the clothes we wear, are ways of caring for the soul.

So finding moments to invest in making yourself feel and look great is always one small contribution to nourishing your soul, too. After all, you are all you've got. Why not make sure you feel and look your best always?

Epilogue

This book first germinated in my mind as a reaction to how shocked I was by the peer pressure women receive even by their closest friends to indulge in one of the ever-popular face fillers that seem trendy and sexy to add to their skin. I listened to countless discussions from my peers that advocate and brag about this new phenomenon that just started after the beginning of the Millennium. I remember writing a column when I was 37 years old weighing the options of Botox to "What would my grandmother think about this?" Should I, too, give in because I was approaching forty?

What seems all too apparent to me – maybe my advertising background has to do something with my theory – is that this is just another way to lure in women and men to spend more of their money, support big companies, plastic surgeon offices and doctors. This book is not against reconstructive surgery with a purpose. This is encouraging you to redirect your steps toward living a more 'soulful life', while embracing your natural beauty first.

While I completely agree that it's fine to look and feel your best, what I don't agree with is changing your actual face structure with a filler to plump it up to appear to look younger, while risking your health.

I am against those needle injections that freeze your face to an extent that you no longer look like your former self. Do you actually want to lose your ability to feel empathy for others, too? These are important facts to consider.

This is an attempt to reason with a person that might be contemplating Botox as a means to fight wrinkles and aging. This is an attempt to implore women to first go within and recognize their soul's wants and needs before masking unhappiness with a 'Barbie doll' look that eventually adds in my opinion, the appearance of lacking emotion and thought.

While writing this book, I have received some sniggers and jeers from some I personally know. *Why?* If it's okay for them to get Botox, then it's okay for me to be against it. I am not alone in my stance. These three amazing actresses – Kate Winslet, Rachel Weisz and Emma Thompson – from the UK have actually formed a group called the "British Anti-Cosmetic Surgery League" with the hopes of helping other women embrace their natural beauty first, too.

I am suggesting easy alternatives that combat stress and to stay healthy without succumbing to believing a two-page spread in *People* magazine advertising this face filler. If you happen to see this ad, you will also see with it the warning disclaimer of all of the side effects, too.

This is not rocket science. Aging is a natural progression that happens to the best of us. After one of my good friends died at the age of 37 from pancreatic cancer without warning, I am here to tell you that a wrinkle on your face is the least of your worries.

What you may not know is that if you are going in for a few Botox injections a year, your face is still going to wrinkle... maybe even far worse with these treatments. So if you can avoid doing this, please do. Please try alternative, natural ways first... just even wearing sunblock every day and washing your face properly before you go to bed. Don't go to sleep with your makeup on... *ever.*

The products I am recommending to you are easy to find. These products have similar ingredients to high-end brands that charge hundreds of dollars for their skin care lines. So make sure you are not wasting your money during a tight economy. Wasting your hundreds of dollars to temporarily achieve a smooth look on your forehead that does not last long-term doesn't make the right equation, does it? That's forgetting the fact it's actually made from a *toxin*. Ask yourself and do the research, how long will this last? How long will this one minute shot that I am spending hundreds of dollars on last? A few months? What will happen when it wears off?

During my mid-thirties I worked as an ad executive selling advertising to local businesses in California. One of my favorite clients ran a medical spa. I just really enjoyed my relationship with this owner. However, I also dreaded that one question, that one push that I knew would always be the crux of our conversation.

"Why don't you try a shot of Botox? You know it's anti-aging, right? How old are you now?"

"Thirty-seven."

"Well, then what are you waiting for?"

"Oh, I work on my expressions. You know I was an actress and learned at an early age to watch my facial expressions. Too many might cause the camera to crack on a close-up."

He usually laughed at that. He thought I was sort of quirky and honestly probably not quite with the modern age woman. Since he was my client I couldn't necessarily tell him that I thought filling my face full of a toxin was something I didn't think my grandmother would agree with or the fact I thought botulism in any form did not belong in my body. Some may think I avoided it because of financial reasons. I definitely could afford Botox, I just didn't want it period.

That was seven years ago. Now I am approaching 42. My birthday is this month. I am edging my way into my mid-forties and do not feel the least bit different. If anything, I am taking a stronger stance against it. I am tired of listening to those ads that are sandwiched in between the nightly news offering a mini-face lift by Debby Boone. I am tired of listening to the Botox clique brag openly about something they haven't even spent time researching yet. This 'clique' is just whimsically going in for their shot without thinking about what this could truly do to their muscles or their skin in even five years. What about ten, what about thirty years? Do think ahead please!

You can still feel youthful at any age if you take proper care of your soul, mind and body. Ask Sophia Loren who just walked the red carpet before the holidays in 2012, and she stole the show even from the younger women that evening. Everyone wanted to know what she did. What was her secret? What was the miracle work that she had done? Sophia Loren just happens to have enough self-confidence and grace within her soul to know that she does not need to alter the structure of her face. This is an example of a woman that I hope to exemplify some day, if I am blessed to live a long and fruitful life. I hope to embrace my natural self and be confident with my real age.

When I was a young model the goal was to stay in shape, sleep well and take care of my skin the natural way. I was told things that stayed with me for a lifetime. Maybe if I had not walked this path, I would not have the courage to be so defiant in my beliefs.

So what are some things to examine when it comes to your looks and your natural self.

Here are some questions to think about:

What am I currently doing to help take care of myself?

Am I on a schedule? Do I actually allow for enough sleep?

Do I take time to nurture my soul so I am in tune with who I am?

Do I know what brings me inner joy?

Do I like my sense of style?

Do I feel like I have a purpose?

Do I care enough about who I am to look within?

Do I try little things to improve my mood and my life every day so I am not just worried about the crinkle between my forehead?

Life is a deeper experience than this. Life is about delving into our deepest thoughts and wishes and watching them materialize in the real world.

If you are living your life like you are letting your age define you, then you are setting yourself up for failure. Think back to my interview with Dr. Patricia Bragg in the Health section. Her attitude, beauty and health are in sync, and she looks and feels amazing. If your inner life with your soul is slightly off, do yourself a favor and do not obsess on tiny lines. This will only cause you more stress and more wrinkles... if you are in fact stressing over aging.

The only alternative is to be six feet under, so start embracing the aging process with a more realistic approach. Like the quote states from the legendary script from *Sunset Boulevard*, there is nothing tragic about being fifty unless are you are trying to be an age you passed up 25 years ago.

At some point I too have been afraid of expiring. You know, like I mentioned as a model, then an actress, and then as a woman. Now I look back and wish I could tell my younger self to *chill out!*

Life is an incredible mystery that we are able to create with our own thoughts and attitude. There is no reason to lie about your age or shave off a few years, *ever*.

Living a truthful existence first with your soul will help you in turn look and feel more radiant.

Some of my tips in the soul/health/beauty sections could be ideas that you are already familiar with on your own path. But make sure to check with yourself and ask yourself these questions often: Are you remembering to take time for yourself? Are you having fun each day? Are you making your health a priority? Are you actively seeking to make who you are on the inside more grounded and sane?

Don't let a little thing like age be the one thing that unravels your confidence. One of the best lines I've ever heard was that one from sexy Suzanne Somers: *"You may not be the youngest person in the room but you can be the sexiest."*

So don't be afraid of your birthdays. *Do* tell the truth about your age. Celebrate them each year. Celebrate who you are with verve and vigor. Don't hide behind a false number. Don't feel ugly because of a wrinkle. And most of all, embrace your natural self. Remember to make small joys happen each day. Most of all, be *you!*

Be yourself.

Be the carefree woman you were during your youth, and release that girl just like you did then. There is no reason to throw in the towel. There is no reason to stop trying to be the best self you can find representing who you are on the inside and out.

I hope that you go forth with a new perspective about your path on your middle age journey. Be confident. Let your years show your spunk, your attitude, and style. Experience silly moments with your friends. 'Remember the three Somethings.' Remember to visualize always and dream. Never settle for less than you were expecting. *So step out onto the center stage of your life and become the star you've always wanted to be.*

Don't sell yourself short or believe you are worth *less* because you are no longer the ripe age of eighteen. So do your best each day to create your moments of joy, discover grand moments like a prizefighter and dare to have some fun anyway... Make one bold step today to be the person you've always wanted to be tomorrow. With that I am letting you know that I am happy to report that being a "Middle Age Beauty" is the best chapter yet. I look forward to the next decade and the next after it. Get creative and dig in each year.

Life can sometimes be short. So don't wait for tomorrow. Act now. Dig into your soul. Dare to discover a rare gem existing within yourself. Discover more dreams. Uplift your thoughts and what else? Have some fun lunches with your girlfriends. Create and be the best you've got. After all, *you* are beautiful inside and out.

Resources/Index

All of the resources for this book were from computer searches online of recent news articles. Personal interviews were given with permission by individuals to be published in this book. You can find more information listed in the index.

Chapter 1 Do Tell the Truth About Your Age
Interview with Dr. Tess Hightower: "About Dr. Tess." <http://www.drtesshightower.com/Dr_Tess_Hightower/Abou t_Dr._Tess.html>.

Chapter 2 Do Say Yes To Your Natural Self. After All, There is Only ONE of You.
Botox is a poison: "Botox injections 'can poison your body'" *Marie Claire*. <http://www.marieclaire.co.uk/news /health/197154/botox-injections-can-poison-your-body.html>.
Side effects from Botox: Staff, Mayo Clinic. "Definition." Mayo Clinic. 06 Feb. 2013. Mayo Foundation for Medical Education and Research. <http://www.mayoclinic.com/health/botox/MY 00078/DSECTION=risks>.
Botox warning to patients and caregivers administering face fillers: "Drugs." <http://www.fda.gov/Drugs/DrugSafety/Post marketDrugSafetyInformationforPatientsandProviders/Drug SafetyInformationforHeathcareProfessionals/ucm143819. htm>.
Canada Botox warning that Botox can spread from original needle injection placement: News, CBC. "Botox Danger - Health Canada confirms - CBC News." CBCnews. 13 Jan. 2009. CBC/Radio Canada. <http://www.cbc.ca/news/story /2009/01/13/botox.html>.
Botox can lessen someone's ability to feel or to feel empathy: Paul, Pamela. "STUDIED: With Botox, Looking Good And

Feeling Less." The New York Times. 19 June 2011. <http://www.nytimes.com/2011/06/19/fashion/bo tox-reduces-the-ability-to-empathize-study-says.html>.

Botox can add to signs of aging by muscle atrophy: "Over Time, Botox May Atrophy Muscles." Sun Sentinel. 23 Feb. 2003. <http://articles.sun-sentinel.com/2003-02-23/health/0302200574_1_botox-muscles-atrophy>.

Chapter 3 Do One Act a Day for Yourself that Brings You Inner Joy

Treasury of Joy and Enthusiasm - Say "YES" To Life by Norman Vincent Peale. 08 Apr. 2013 <http://www.vanguardbooks.com/browsetitle.php?isbn=8122203736>.

Chapter 4 Important Questions for the Soul

Interview with MJ Rolek: FunZen Bakery. <http://funzen bakery.blogspot.com/>.

Chapter 5 Visualize What You Want to Be

John Huston story reference from: John Huston: *The Man, the Movies, the Maverick*. IMDb. IMDb.com. <http://www.im db.com/title/tt0095408/>.

Chapter 6 Find Time To Make New Friends

Julie/Julia Reference: *"Julie & Julia."* IMDb. IMDb.com. 08 Apr. 2013 <http://www.imdb.com/title/tt1135503/>.

"Julie Powell Books." <http://juliepowellbooks.com/>.

Riding, Alan. "Becoming Julia Child." *The New York Times*. 28 May 2006. <http://www.nytimes.com/2006/05/28/books/review/28riding.html>.

Chapter 7 Moments Like Seinfeld

Seinfeld like moment is inspired by the American television sitcom that originally aired on NBC from July 5, 1989, to May

14, 1998. The show was created by Jerry Seinfeld and Larry David. It lasted nine seasons, and is now in syndication. "Seinfeld - Official Site." <http://www.sonypictures.com/tv /shows/seinfeld/>.

"Jerry Seinfeld - Personal Archives." Jerry Seinfeld. <http:// www.jerryseinfeld.com/>.

"Larry David" - "Imdb." Wikipedia. 04 Wikimedia Foundation. http://www.imdb.com/name/nm0202970/?ref_=sr_1

Chapter 8 Are you in Touch With Your Leadership Skills?

Interview with Dr. Anthony F. Smith: "Dr. Anthony F. Smith." <http://www.dranthonyfsmith.com/about.html>.

Chapter 9 Be Optimistic with Your Thoughts

"Norman Vincent Peale Home Page." <http://normanvincent peale.wwwhubs.com/>.

Chapter 11 Create a 'Rocky Like Moment' Three Times a Week

"Sylvester Stallone." <http://www.sylvesterstallone.com/>

Rocky. IMDb. IMDb.com.

http://www.imdb.com/title/tt0075148/

"Rocky (film series)." Wikipedia. Wikimedia Foundation. <http://en.wikipedia.org/wiki/Rocky_(film_series)>.

Chapter 13 Rescue a Pet

"Health Talk." <http://www.health.umn.edu/healthtalk/2012 /07/09/what-has-nine-lives-and-makes-you-live-longer/>.

"Our President-Mike Arms." Our President. <http://www.animal center.org/about_hwac/our_president.aspx>.

"The Dog Who Helped A Boy To Speak." CBSNews. 11 Feb. 2009. CBS Interactive. <http://www.cbsnews.com/8301-500617_162-3940707.html>.

Chapter 15 Meditation verses Botox

"Worst Foodborne Illness Outbreaks in U.S. History." <http://www.healthline.com/health-slideshow/worst-foodborne-illness-outbreaks>.

Crosta, Peter. "What Is Botox? How Does Botox Work?" Medical News Today. 24 July 2009. MediLexicon International. <http://www.medicalnewstoday.com/articles/158647.php>.

FunZen Bakery. 08 Apr. 2013 <http://funzenbakery.blogspot.com/>. M.J. Rolek

Chapter 16 Your Health

Lovett, Edward. "Most Models Meet Criteria for Anorexia, Size 6 Is Plus Size: Magazine." *ABC News*. ABC News Network. <http://abcnews.go.com/blogs/headlines/2012/01/most-models-meet-criteria-for-anorexia-size-6-is-plus-size-magazine/>.

"Bragg *Apple Cider Vinegar* Book, Bragg Live Foods, Bragg Apple Cider Vinegar, Bragg Liquid Aminos, Systemic Enzymes, Bragg Live Organic Food Products, Patricia Bragg, Paul Bragg, Bragg Organic Olive Oil, Bragg Salad Dressings, Bragg Seasonings, Bragg Health Products." Bragg Apple Cider Vinegar Book, Bragg Live Foods, <http://bragg.com/books/acv_excerpt .html>.

"The 17 Day Diet." The 17 Day Diet. <http://www.the17 daydiet.com/>. Dr. Mike Moreno

Chapter 17 Life Giving Molecule: Melatonin

"CSB Faculty." Faculty of the Dept of Cellular and Structural Biology. <http://www.uthscsa.edu/csb/faculty/reiter.asp>.

MELATONIN." <http://www.stensrude.com/me latonin.html>.

Chapter 18 Apple Cider Vinegar Nature's Healing Miracle

"Bragg *Apple Cider Vinegar* Book, Bragg Live Foods, Bragg Apple Cider Vinegar, Bragg Liquid Aminos, Systemic Enzymes,

Bragg Live Organic Food Products, Patricia Bragg, Paul Bragg, Bragg Organic Olive Oil, Bragg Salad Dressings, Bragg Seasonings, Bragg Health Products." <http://bragg.com/books/acv_excerpt.html>.

Chapter 20 Weigh In With Yourself

"Simon & Schuster." Simon & Schuster <http://authors.simonand schuster.com/Dr-Mike-Moreno/83851483?intcmp=l_fl>.

Chapter 21 Easy Diet Tips and Food Suggestions That Can Help You Manage Your Weight

"What is the difference between sweet potatoes and yams?" Everyday Mysteries: Fun Science Facts from the Library of Congress. http://www.loc.gov/rr/scitech/mysteries/sweet potato.html

08 Apr. 2013 <http://www.whfoods.com/genpage.php?tna me=foodspice>.

"Archive for April, 2011." Door to Door Organics Chicago RSS. <https://blog.doortodoororganics.com/chicago/2011/04/>.

"Best Healthy Foods You Aren't Eating: Greek Yogurt, Canned Tomatoes, and More." WebMD. <http://www.webmd.com /diet/features/best-foods-you-are-not-eating?page=2>

"Food & Wellness." Fox News Magazine. <http://magazine .foxnews.com/food-wellness/truth-about-diet-drinks>

"How to Lose Weight on an Oatmeal Diet." LIVESTRONG.COM. <http://www.livestrong.com/article/31401-lose-weight-oatmeal-diet/>.

Chapter 22 Goodbye Sophistication, Hello Smaller Waistline

Sideways. IMDb. IMDb.com. <http://www.imdb.com/title/tt03 75063/>.

"The Health Effects of Alcohol." About.com Alcoholism. <http://alcoholism.about.com/od/health/Effects_of_Alcohol_ Health_Effects_of_Alcohol.htm>.

Centers for Disease Control and Prevention. <http://www.cdc.gov/>.

"Nutritional Information Facts, Glycemic Index, and Zone Blocks." Nutritional Information Facts, Glycemic Index, and Zone Blocks. <http://www.formulazone.com/Help.asp?TID=ILUP>.

Chapter 23 The One Shot You Need: Vitamin B Shots

"Benefits of Vitamin B12 Injections." LIVESTRONG.COM. <http://www.livestrong.com/article/109578-benefits-vitamin-b12-injections/>.

"IV Nutrition / B12 Shots." Myer's Cocktail. <http://www.naturedockelly.com/wp/services/ivnutrition>.

Chapter 24 Why 15 Minutes or Less Can Help You Work Out More.

"GEICO's Crazy Ad Strategy Breaks the Rules." The Financial Brand Marketing Insights for Banks Credit Unions RSS. <http://thefinancialbrand.com/9663/geico-gecko-caveman-kash-tv-commercials/>.

Gorman, Christine. "Walk, Don't Run." *Time.* <http://www.time.com/time/magazine/article/0,9171,1001678,00.html>.

"Olivia Newton-John: Let's Get Physical." IMDb. IMDb.com. <http://www.imdb.com/title/tt0283520/>.

Staff, Mayo Clinic. "Walking: Trim your waistline, improve your health." Mayo Clinic. 18 Dec. 2010. Mayo Foundation for Medical Education and Research. <http://www.mayoclinic.com/health/walking/HQ01612>.

Chapter 25 Omega 3 and Fish Oil Pills

"Omega-3 Fish Oil Supplements: Benefits, Side Effects, and Uses." WebMD. 01 Mar. 2013. <http://www.webmd.com/hypertension-high-blood-pressure/guide/omega-3-fishoil-supplements-for-high-blood-pressure>.

"Home." <http://www.nutritionenergy.com/main/page_our_
nutritionists_lauren_antonucci_ms_rd_cssd_cde_cdn.html>.

Chapter 26 Your Beauty

"Beauty." Definition of in Oxford Dictionaries (US English) (US).
<http://oxforddictionaries.com/us/definition/american
_english/beauty>.

Chapter 28 My Secret Weapon in Fighting Wrinkles

"Jennifer Aniston's £1 beauty secret: Actress smooths Vaseline
under her eyes to look flawless at 43." *Mail Online.*
<http://www.dailymail.co.uk/femail/article-2157570/Jennifer-
Anistons-1-beauty-secret-Actress-43-smooths-Vaseline-eyes-
maintain-youthful-look.html>.
"How to Use Preparation H for Wrinkles." LIVESTRONG.COM.
<http://www.livestrong.com/article/16489-use-preparation-h-
wrinkles/>.

Chapter 32 ICON Chic

"Actress Audrey Hepburn dies." History.com. A&E Television
Networks. <http://www.history.com/this-day-in-history/act
ress-audrey-hepburn-dies>.
"*Two for the Road.*" IMDb. IMDb.com. <http://www.imdb.
com/title/tt0062407/>.

Chapter 33 Think PINK!

"How choosing the right clothes can make you look 15 YEARS
younger." *Mail Online.* <http://www.dailymail.co.uk/femail
/article-2172618/How-choosing-right-clothes-make-look-15-
years-younger.html>.

Chapter 34 Keep Fashion Simple

"*When Harry Met Sally...*" IMDb. IMDb.com. <http://www.
imdb.com/title/tt0098635/>.

Chapter 35 Beauty Product Tips

All products listed in this chapter can be found: "Amazon.com: Online Shopping for Electronics, Apparel, Computers, Books, DVDs & more." <http://www.amazon.com/>.

**AYNI
BOOKS**

"Ayni" is a Quechua word meaning "reciprocity" – sharing, giving and receiving – whatever you give out comes back to you. To be in Ayni is to be in balance, harmony and right relationship with oneself and nature, of which we are all an intrinsic part. Complementary and Alternative approaches to health and well-being essentially follow a holistic model, within which one is given support and encouragement to move towards a state of balance, true health and wholeness, ultimately leading to the awareness of one's unique place in the Universal jigsaw of life – Ayni, in fact.